Orthofacial Surgery

Federico Hernández-Alfaro
Adaia Valls Ontañón
Editors

Orthofacial Surgery

Aesthetic & Functional Surgery of the Facial Skeleton and Mask

Springer

Editors
Federico Hernández-Alfaro
Department of Oral and Maxillofacial Surgery
International University of Catalonia
Barcelona, Spain

Adaia Valls Ontañón
Department of Oral and Maxillofacial Surgery
International University of Catalonia
Barcelona, Spain

ISBN 978-3-031-76184-3 ISBN 978-3-031-76185-0 (eBook)
https://doi.org/10.1007/978-3-031-76185-0

This Springer imprint is published by the registered company Springer Nature Switzerland AG
The registered company address is: Gewerbestrasse 11, 6330 Cham, Switzerland

Foreword

Reflecting to the past, I realized I met Federico Hernández-Alfaro for the first time at the 20th National Congress of the Spanish Association of Oral and Maxillofacial Surgery (OMFS) in Bilbao, Spain, in 2009. It was Domingo Martin, orthodontist from San Sebastian, who presented me at that time to Federico and his "bro" Mirco Raffaini. Both of them should be considered the pioneers of "orthofacial surgery" worldwide.

Since then, I had the pleasure to meet Federico at many scientific meetings and nice social events overall in the world and we became close friends. I am personally very proud that he proposed me to not only become an associate professor of his OMFS Department, Universitat Internacional de Catalunya, Spain, but also co-direct the first Spanish European PhD thesis by his resident and my fellow Raquel Guijarro Martínez on "Cone-Beam Computerized Tomography (CBCT) Evaluation of the Upper Airway in the Context of Orthognathic Surgery", May 2014.

Orthognathic surgery has been well developed in the past in the 1980s and 1990s to treat different types of maxillofacial deformities both functionally and aesthetically. In the new millennium, treatment strategies however went far beyond occlusal correction. The advent of CBCT, 3D virtual planning, minimally invasive (MI) surgical techniques, and simultaneous ancillary surgical techniques to enhance the aesthetics of the overlying soft tissue mask has definitely changed "orthognathic surgery" into "orthofacial surgery".

With "Orthofacial Surgery" by the editors Federico Hernández-Alfaro and Adaia Valls-Ontañón, the reader has a marvellous manuscript towards aesthetic and functional surgery of the facial skeleton and the overlying soft tissue mask in their hands. It provides a comprehensive, evidence-based overview of the latest advancements in orthognathic and orthofacial surgery, supported by state-of-the-art publications. It describes in a highly detailed way all aspects of "orthofacial surgery" in 15 consecutive chapters: Facial Diagnosis (Chap. 1); The Long Face (Chap. 2); The Short Face (Chap. 3); Transverse Problems (Chap. 4); Facial Asymmetry (Chap. 5); Surgical Orthodontics (Chap. 6); Clear Aligner Therapy in Orthognathic Surgery (Chap. 7); Three-Dimensional Planning in Orthofacial Surgery (Chap. 8); Minimally Invasive Surgery of the Maxilla (Chap. 9); Minimally Invasive Surgery of the Mandible (Chap. 10); Surgery of the Chin (Chap. 11); Simultaneous Bimaxillary Surgery and Rhinoplasty and Evolving Concepts in Orthofacial Surgery (Chap. 12); Ancillary Procedures in Orthofacial

Surgery (Chap. 13); Peroperative Surgical Management and Recommendations (Chap. 14); and finally, Airway and Skeletal Surgery (Chap. 15).

Both authors need to be congratulated on their standardized and systematized approach to "orthofacial surgery", which is truly unique.

Professor Federico Hernández-Alfaro is a distinguished and world-renowned authority in the field of OMFS. His profound scientific insights and innovative surgical treatment strategies have firmly established him as a pioneer in "orthofacial surgery". His extensive body of evidence-based research, groundbreaking peer-reviewed publications, and many national and international lectures serves as essential references for both established specialists and young "NextGen" surgeons who will further shape the future of OMFS. Our shared passion for innovation, precision, and interdisciplinary collaboration has pushed a relationship of mutual respect, marked by continuous academic and clinical exchange. Moreover, and last but not least, Federico Hernández-Alfaro is an inspiring mentor to the profession of both surgeons (including myself) and orthodontists. This book marks an absolute and important new milestone and is an absolute "must-read"!

I hereby extend my deepest appreciation to Professor Hernández-Alfaro for his tireless contributions to the OMFS and orthodontic field and I am more than confident that this book will set a new benchmark in the literature on orthognathic and orthofacial surgery. I wish the reader an enriching and inspiring journey through the pages of this outstanding and brilliant work.

Gwen R. J. Swennen

Division of Maxillofacial Surgery
and Facial Plastic Surgery,
Department of Surgery
AZ Sint-Jan Brugge AV
Bruges, Belgium
February 2025

Preface: From Orthognathic to Orthofacial Surgery

A decade ago, 90% of my surgical patients with dentofacial deformities were referred by orthodontists for a combined ortho-surgical approach to manage malocclusions. Today, 70% of our patients initially visit our office with concerns primarily about facial aesthetics and airway issues.

The term "orthognathic surgery", referring to skeletal surgery aimed at correcting malocclusions, is now obsolete. In its place, a new concept has emerged, signalling a paradigm shift in the contemporary management of facial deformities.

"Orthofacial surgery" is defined as aesthetic and functional surgery of the facial skeleton and its overlying soft tissues. This approach extends beyond traditional "orthognathic surgery" and "facial aesthetic surgery". Previously, orthognathic surgery focused primarily on correcting altered occlusions through 3D repositioning of the maxilla and mandible. Conversely, facial aesthetic surgery primarily deals with the management of facial soft tissues and often focuses on facial rejuvenation.

Modern orthodontics can often successfully correct malocclusions and achieve a proper bite; however, facial aesthetics and airway concerns have become major factors for many patients.

Orthofacial surgery aims to normalize the facial skeleton and the overlying soft tissues. It requires surgeons to be comprehensively trained in order to adopt a holistic approach to facial issues.

There are three primary reasons why patients might seek orthofacial surgery. Firstly, aesthetic concerns often involve the facial structure—including the maxilla, mandible, chin, nose, and/or malar areas—and the soft tissue mask. Secondly, patients often present with altered dental occlusions caused by abnormal sizes or positions of the maxilla or mandible; aesthetic concerns are almost always concurrent. Thirdly, an increasing number of patients suffer from obstructive sleep apnea syndrome (OSAS), which is often poorly managed with continuous airway pressure devices. Maxillo-mandibular advancement has proven to be the only curative method for patients with moderate and severe OSAS.

The management of dentofacial deformities has undergone significant changes recently. Clinical aesthetic diagnosis has replaced traditional cephalometric approaches in facial surgical planning: it is no longer just about measurements but about proportions and the subjective perception of beauty. Additionally, 3D planning enables the precise execution of the surgical plan in the operating room, minimizing the need for intraoperative improvisation.

Minimally invasive surgical principles have also transformed the field, fostering an empathic approach that reduces extensive surgical exposure and soft tissue disruption. The principle of "less is more" aptly describes this new approach.

Thanks to these innovations, "orthognathic surgery" is presently considered to be an outdated concept. Meanwhile, a new philosophy of "orthofacial surgery" has emerged. In subsequent chapters, we will explore all the procedures associated with orthofacial surgery and various clinical scenarios.

Barcelona, Spain Federico Hernández-Alfaro

Contents

1 **Facial Diagnosis** . . . 1
Federico Hernández-Alfaro

2 **Vertical Problems: The Long Face** . . . 5
Federico Hernández-Alfaro

3 **The Short Face** . . . 15
Federico Hernández-Alfaro

4 **Transverse Problems** . . . 29
Federico Hernández-Alfaro

5 **Facial Asymmetry** . . . 35
Federico Hernández-Alfaro, Orion-Luiz Haas-Junior, and Adaia Valls Ontañón

6 **Surgical Orthodontics** . . . 51
Juan Carlos Pérez Varela, Miriam López Vila, and Laura González García

7 **Clear Aligner Therapy in Orthognathic Surgery** . . . 63
Oriol Quevedo Pou, Fernando de la Iglesia Beyme, and Ariadna Pamies Parejo

8 **Three-Dimensional Planning in Orthofacial Surgery** . . . 75
Orion-Luiz Haas-Junior

9 **Minimally Invasive Surgery of the Maxilla** . . . 87
Federico Hernández-Alfaro

10 **Minimally Invasive Surgery of the Mandible** . . . 97
Adaia Valls Ontañón and Federico Hernández-Alfaro

11 **Surgery of the Chin** . . . 109
Adaia Valls Ontañón and Federico Hernández-Alfaro

12 **Simultaneous Bimaxillary Surgery and Rhinoplasty: Evolving Concepts in Orthofacial Surgery** . . . 115
Mirco Raffaini and Francesco Arcuri

13 Ancillary Procedures in Orthofacial Surgery: Malarplasty, Lipofilling, Bichectomy, and Jaw Angles 127
Tulsi Roy and Derek M. Steinbacher

14 Peroperative Surgical Management and Recommendations . . . 139
Adaia Valls Ontañón and Orion-Luiz Haas-Junior

15 Airway and Skeletal Surgery 147
Adaia Valls Ontañón

Facial Diagnosis

1

Federico Hernández-Alfaro

1.1 Why Not Cephalometry?

Planning in orthognathic surgery has been and remains an open issue. We have evolved from two-dimensional (2D) classical cephalometric hard-tissue planning to 2D soft-tissue planning [1] and finally to three-dimensional (3D) and hard- and soft-tissue evaluation [2, 3]. In all cases, the goal has been to establish normative data that could be used by clinicians to diagnose and plan the treatment of dentofacial deformities.

There are two important limitations. Most of the "classical" cephalometric analyses reflect a norm derived from a limited number of average individuals not necessarily attractive and with normal occlusions. On the other hand, when different cephalometric analyses are applied to a particular individual, the diagnosis and thus the treatment plan may vary between them [4]. These analyses can at best enhance orthodontic diagnosis and treatment planning, but they are used mainly for descriptive purposes. Individual tracings are compared to an average facial pattern, and the difference between them requires considerable interpretation.

F. Hernández-Alfaro (✉)
Department of Oral and Maxillofacial Surgery, International University of Catalonia, Barcelona, Spain
e-mail: h.alfaro@uic.es

The studies of Farkas et al. [5] and posterior developments by authors such as Holdaway [6, 7], Merrifield [8], and Arnett et al. [9, 10] brought attention to the soft tissues (facial mask) in aesthetic diagnosis and planning.

For patients with dentofacial deformities, Sarver et al. [11] introduced the concept of centripetal construction of the face, whereby the soft tissues should guide skeletal correction.

Arnett must be mentioned for being the first author to truly systematize a comprehensive facial soft tissue analysis in both the frontal and sagittal planes. However, the normative data for the analysis of Arnett were extracted from a rather small sample of "attractive" subjects, according to the author. On the other hand, his facial measures are related to a vertical line through the subnasale. In our experience, this line does not constitute a stable reference, considering that a great majority of disharmonic surgical patients have varying degrees of maxillary hypoplasia (95%). These circumstances prevent the use of this line as an absolute reference.

In sum, no current cephalometric analysis can be used as an absolute road map for facial planning—the main reason being that no algorithm has been able so far to include a big enough population of normal/attractive individuals segmented by race, age, sex, geographical location, etc.

By no means am I condemning cephalometric analyses. They are perfect to analyze dentoskel-

F. Hernández-Alfaro, A. Valls Ontañón (eds.), *Orthofacial Surgery*,
https://doi.org/10.1007/978-3-031-76185-0_1

etal relations, hard/soft tissue relations, performing superimpositions, monitoring growth, evaluating relapse, etc.

My personal philosophy can be summarized as follows: "Frontal (symmetry) and occlusal parameters are objective and can be measured. Sagittal (vertical and anteroposterior) parameters are subjective and constitute the artistic part of this specialty, which, as from now, will be referred to as orthofacial surgery".

Also, when it comes to facial planning, we are not focusing on measurements or absolute dimensions but on harmony and proportions.

In the rest of this chapter, I will try to describe my personal approach to facial planning.

1.2 Two Rules of Facial Harmony

At this point, one might think that losing cephalometry as a strict guide for facial diagnosis and planning could be like navigating an uncharted sea. The truth is that it is indeed somehow that way. However, there are several aspects that should be considered when planning orthofacial surgery.

According to our personal "*3D Facial Aesthetic Design*," a harmonious face should abide with two rules which can be summarized as follows: symmetry and facial projection (i.e., vertical, transverse, and anteroposterior proportions). These generic concepts must accompany all therapeutic efforts in facial surgery. All faces which any of us may consider attractive include both of these rules.

1.2.1 Symmetry

Harmonious faces are symmetrical. But on the other hand, completely symmetrical faces do not exist. The goal should be to achieve enough symmetry for the patient to be perceived as symmetric by himself and by peers. We have a specific chapter dealing with the diagnosis and management of facial asymmetries. Three-dimensional planning has obviously contributed to better understand problems in the frontal plane and to more precisely evaluate levels of asymmetry in the face (Fig. 1.1).

1.2.2 Facial Projection

1.2.2.1 Facial Anterior Projection (FAP)

If we set a coronal plane through the soft tissue nasion with the patient at rest (natural head position), all elements of a harmonious face should basically be projected in front of this plane. This obviously depends on the relative projection of the maxilla and mandible and also involves the nose, lips, and chin support. We will later analyze

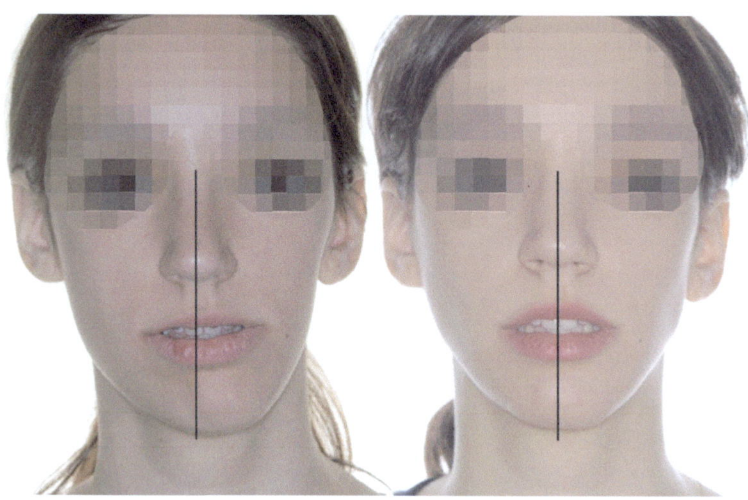

Fig. 1.1 Symmetry is a binary concept. Perfect symmetry, however, does not exist in human nature. We need to achieve enough symmetry for the patient to be perceived as symmetrical by him/herself and by others

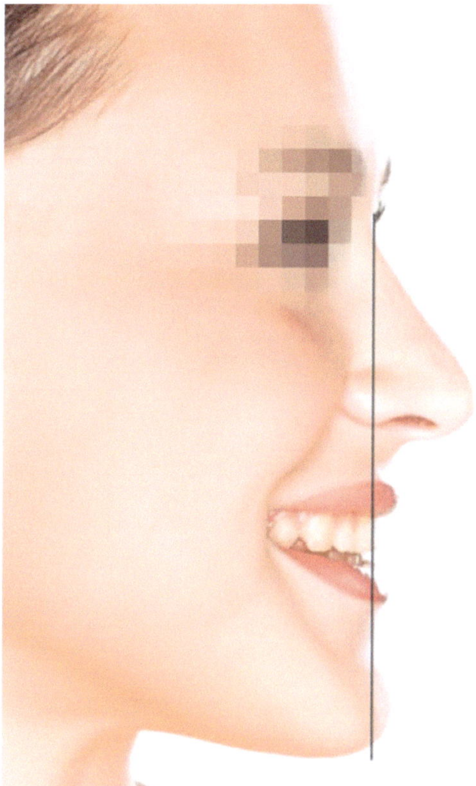

Fig. 1.2 The upper incisor to soft-tissue plane or "Barcelona Line" is an absolute reference when it comes to determine an appropriate anterior facial projection

how we use this specific soft-tissue plane (STP) as an absolute reference in facial planning [1] (Fig. 1.2).

1.2.2.2 Facial Vertical Projection (FVP)

Vertical problems should not be analyzed cephalometrically. A face could impress us as being short, normal, or long, irrespective of any measures or tracings. Once we get this impression, identification of the cause for that impression will give us the clues to plan its correction (Fig. 1.3).

1.2.2.3 Facial Transverse Projection (FTP)

This concept has an occlusal component and a facial one. Transverse maxillomandibular discrepancy has important occlusal implications and will be dealt with in a separate chapter.

Transverse proportions between the middle and lower thirds of the face are also paramount to facial beauty and will be covered later in this book.

1.2.2.4 Soft-Tissue Support

This concept somehow summarizes and is a consequence of the previous concept. No matter how

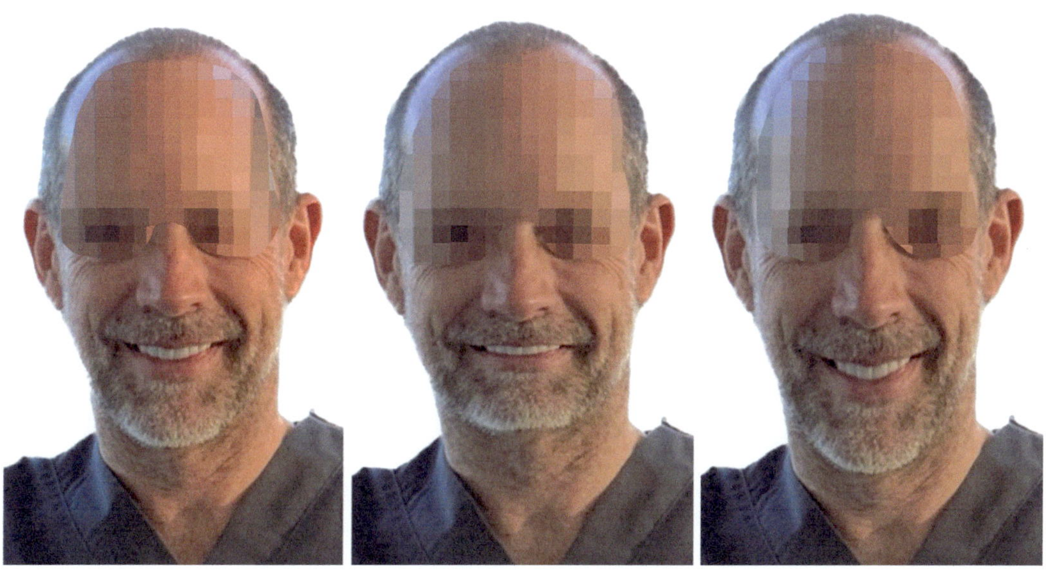

Fig. 1.3 The perception of "short" or "long" is not always related to the proportion of the facial thirds

we plan a face, its volume at the end of surgery must be equal to or greater than the preoperative volume. The reason for this is to maintain or (even better) increase support for the facial mask. The opposite results in premature aging. This means that contracting or posteriorly repositioning some skeletal parts has to be compensated by the expansion or anterior repositioning of others. Besides aesthetic reasons, there is a fundamental functional reason: skeletal contraction might provoke reduction of the airway and thus sleep apnea.

It is obvious that most dentofacial deformities present different combinations of problems, but at any rate, all five traits should be collected and implemented when planning for facial skeletal surgery (orthofacial surgery).

In the end, when diagnosing and planning facial correction, we have to consider that occlusal and frontal (symmetry) problems can be accurately objectivized, whereas sagittal ones cannot, and should remain in the subjective (artistic) arena.

References

1. Hernández-Alfaro F. Upper incisor to Soft Tissue Plane (UI-STP): a new reference for diagnosis and planning in dentofacial deformities. Med Oral Patol Oral Cir Bucal. 2010;15(5):e779–81.
2. Paredes de Sousa Gil A, Guijarro-Martínez R, Haas OL Jr, Hernández-Alfaro F. Three-dimensional analysis of nasolabial soft tissue changes after Le Fort I osteotomy: a systematic review of the literature. Int J Oral Maxillofac Surg. 2019;48(9):1185–200.
3. Incrapera AK, Kau CH, English JD, McGrory K, Sarver DM. Soft tissue images from cephalograms compared with those from a 3D surface acquisition system. Angle Orthod. 2010;80:58–64.
4. Wylie GA, Fish LC, Epker BN. Cephalometrics: a comparison of five analyses currently used in the diagnosis of dentofacial deformities. Int J Adult Orthodon Orthognath Surg. 1987;2:15–36.
5. Farkas LG, Eiben OG, Sivkov S, Tompson B, Katic MJ, Forrest CR. Anthropometric measurements of the facial framework in adulthood: age-related changes in eight age categories in 600 healthy white North Americans of European ancestry from 16 to 90 years of age. J Craniofac Surg. 2004;15:288–98.
6. Holdaway RA. A soft-tissue cephalometric analysis and its use in orthodontic treatment planning. Part I. Am J Orthod. 1983;84(1–28):5.
7. Holdaway RA. A soft-tissue cephalometric analysis and its use in orthodontic treatment planning. Part II. Am J Orthod. 1984;85:279–93.
8. Merrifield LL. The profile line as an aid in critically evaluating facial esthetics. Am J Orthod. 1966;52:804–22.
9. Arnett GW, Bergman RT. Facial keys to orthodontic diagnosis and treatment planning. Part I. Am J Orthod Dentofacial Orthop. 1993;103:299–312.
10. Arnett GW, Bergman RT. Facial keys to orthodontic diagnosis and treatment planning. Part II. Am J Orthod Dentofacial Orthop. 1993;103:395–411.
11. Sarver DM, Rousso DR. Plastic surgery combined with orthodontic and orthognathic procedures. Am J Orthod Dentofacial Orthop. 2004;126:305–7.

2 Vertical Problems: The Long Face

Federico Hernández-Alfaro

2.1 Diagnosis

The diagnosis of a long face follows exactly the same sequence as that described for a short face [1]. Once we get the "impression" of a long face, we need to break down the problem, and again there are four traits, alone or combined, which can give that impression: vertical excess of the maxilla, vertical excess of the chin, open bite, and narrow face (Fig. 2.1).

Correction of a long face entails a therapeutic dilemma, however: we should theoretically shorten the face, but this inevitably would provoke loss of soft tissue support and thus premature facial aging.

2.1.1 How Can We Solve This Conflict?

There are basically two strategies: first, to always undershorten the face, meaning staying on the "long" side, and, second, to project the face anteriorly, thus maintaining adequate support for the facial soft tissue mask.

F. Hernández-Alfaro (✉)
Department of Oral and Maxillofacial Surgery, International University of Catalonia, Barcelona, Spain
e-mail: h.alfaro@uic.es

A long face needs to stay long. If you check on the Internet for models, actors, and appealing harmonious faces, you will realize that most attractive individuals have the lower third of the face which is longer than the middle third.

When I am planning for correction of a long face, I like to vertically undercorrect the maxilla, limiting my impactions and, particularly in young women, maintaining some degree of lip incompetence. Besides preserving soft-tissue support, this strategy will avoid excessive lip competence or the absence of incisal display some years down the road. The bottom line is that when correcting a long face, it is more about changing the components and correcting negative traits than about actually shortening the face (Fig. 2.2).

There is a second strategy to overcome the therapeutic dilemma which appears when shortening a face but still willing to maintain an adequate soft-tissue support. It consists of projecting the face forward. More specifically, whenever we need to either impact the maxilla, close an open bite, or vertically reduce the chin, we need to compensate this vertical reduction with anterior repositioning of the maxillomandibular complex (Fig. 2.3). This forward repositioning in our protocol follows the Barcelona Line as an absolute reference [2] (Fig. 2.4).

The typical and more prevalent "long face syndrome" usually presents with an open bite, maxillary excess, and a posteriorly rotated

F. Hernández-Alfaro, A. Valls Ontañón (eds.), *Orthofacial Surgery*,
https://doi.org/10.1007/978-3-031-76185-0_2

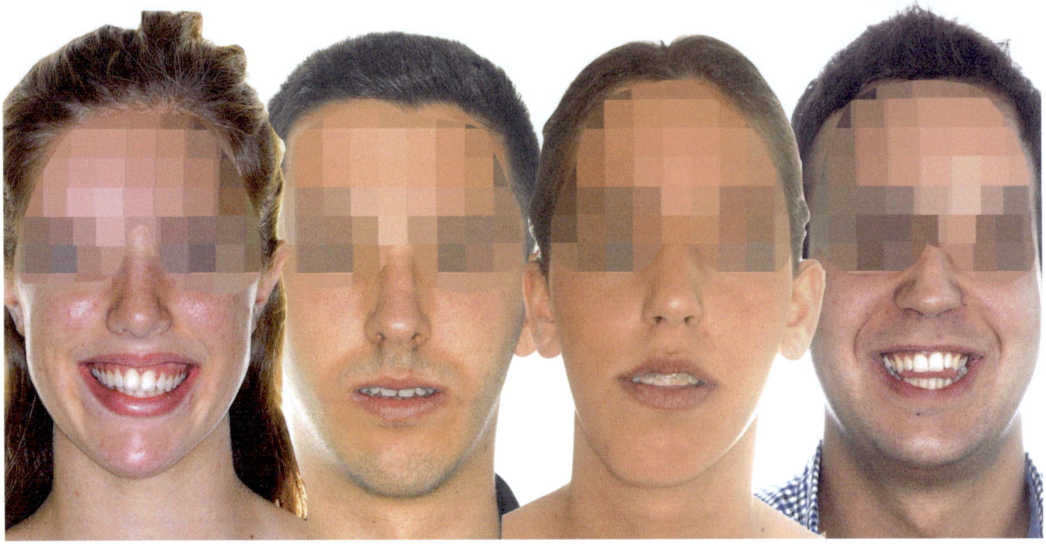

Fig. 2.1 A long face can be the result of one of the following traits, alone or combined: vertical maxillary hyperplasia, vertical chin excess, narrow face, and open bite

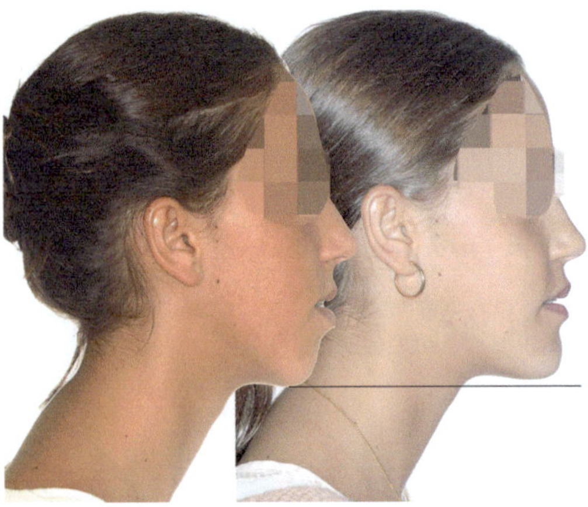

Fig. 2.2 Pre- and postoperative view illustrating that a long face should stay "long"

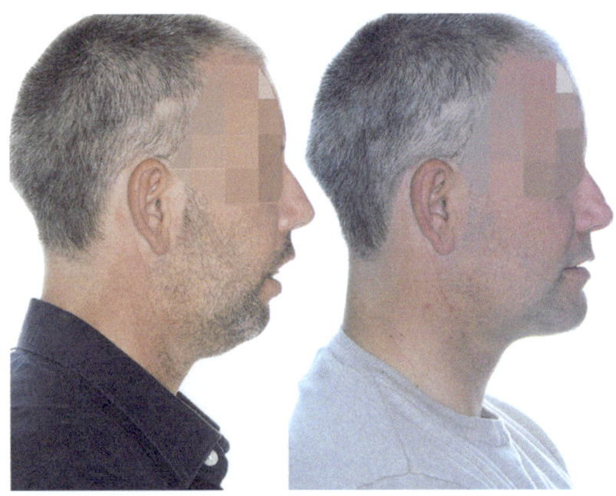

Fig. 2.3 Shortening of the face should be accompanied by anterior projection (face push) to preserve soft-tissue support

mandible [1]. It can be accompanied by Angle class II (Fig. 2.5) or class III occlusion. In addition to the aforementioned characteristics, a class III long face usually presents with a hypoplastic maxilla in the anteroposterior dimension (Fig. 2.6).

In contrast to what we have mentioned in relation to short faces, long face management typically includes counterclockwise rotation of the occlusal plane. The reason for this is the fact that most long face patients present with a posteriorly rotated mandible, which provokes lengthening of the face and a lack of jawline and chin–neck definition (Fig. 2.7).

General therapeutic goals in long face management could be summarized as follows:

- To achieve class I occlusion and adequate overbite, correct incisal exposure, anterior projection of the face, definition of the labiomental fold, and the maintenance of soft-tissue support.

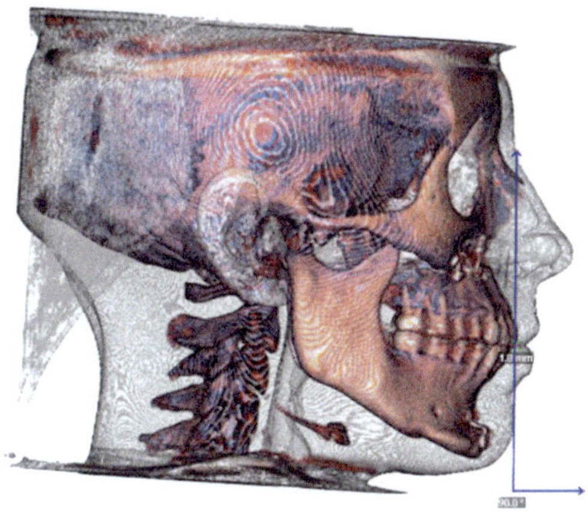

Fig. 2.4 Forward repositioning of the maxillomandibular complex following the Barcelona Line as an absolute reference

Closing the open bite tends to be the most important occlusal goal in long face patients. The orthodontist needs to evaluate transverse and vertical intra-arch problems. When a pronounced curve of Spee is present in the maxilla, orthodontic preparation should proceed with a two-level segmental preparation [3, 4]. With the aid of sectional or utility arches, a step should be generated between laterals and cuspids. Then, upper arch leveling is achieved surgically by segmenting the maxilla [5] (Fig. 2.8a and b).

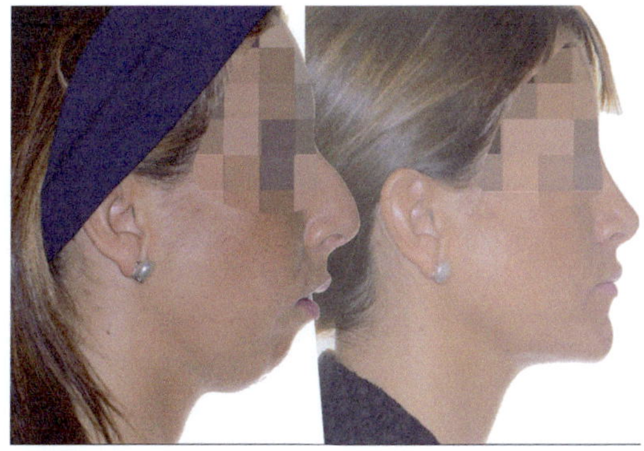

Fig. 2.5 Counterclockwise rotation of the occlusal plane is indicated in most cases of long face

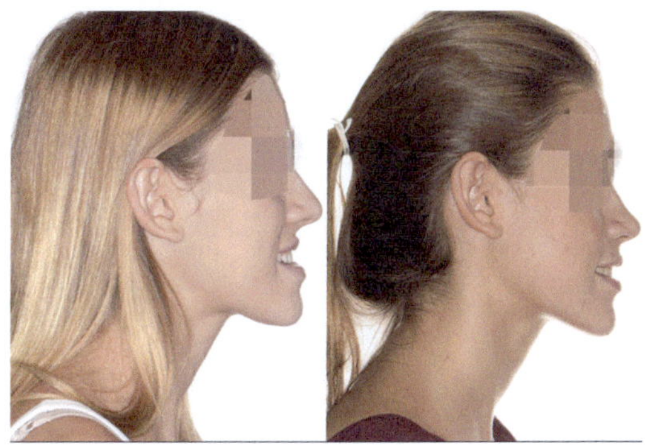

Fig. 2.6 Class III occlusion is also frequently associated with a long face and should be managed with the same principles

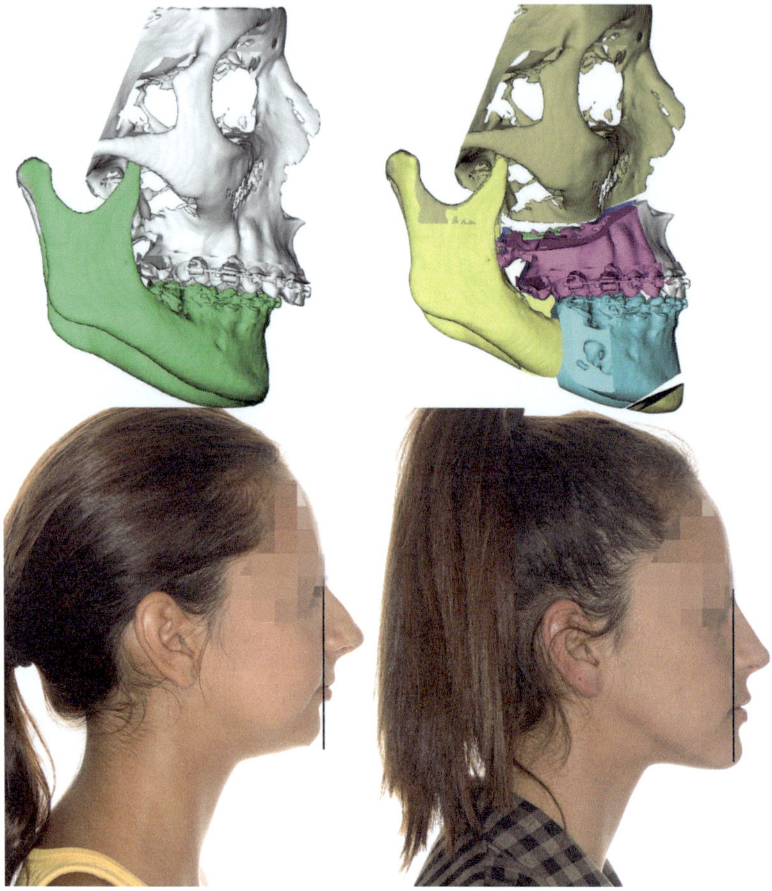

Fig. 2.7 The Barcelona Line serves as an absolute reference for anterior maxillomandibular repositioning

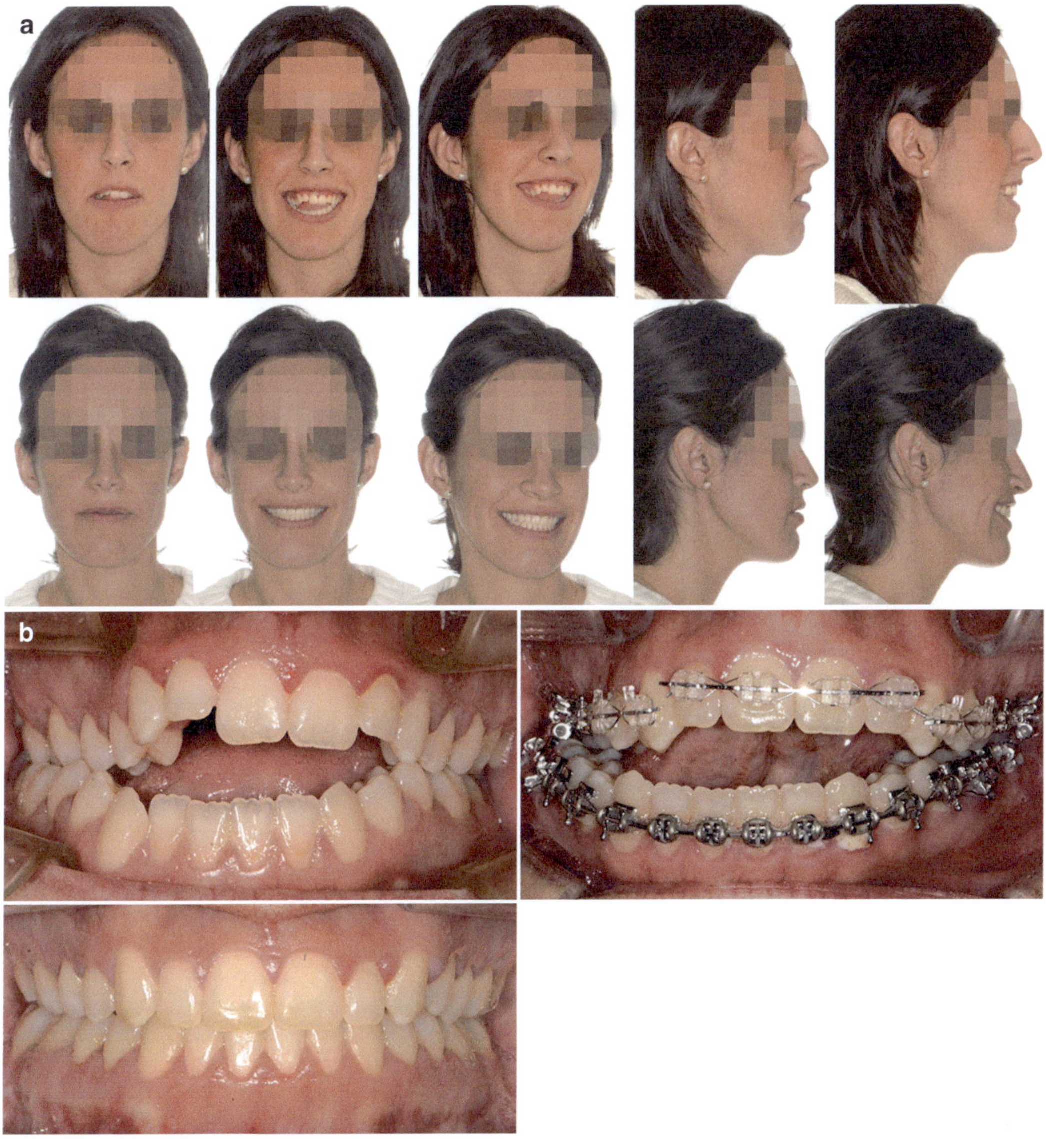

Fig. 2.8 (**a** and **b**) Long face secondary to vertical maxillary excess and open bite, corrected with double jaw surgery

2.2 Gummy Smile

This is one of the most prevalent characteristics of a long face [6]. When analyzing a gummy or gingival smile, it is of utmost importance to establish an adequate differential diagnosis and rule out the possible altered passive eruption as well as lip hypermobility [7, 8]. The former is managed with periodontal surgery and the latter with botulinum toxin [6, 9].

The third and probably the most frequent cause of gummy smile is vertical maxillary excess.

Surgical management of the smile basically consists of either impacting, downgrafting, or leveling the maxilla (Fig. 2.9) in order to modify incisal/gingival exposure, both at rest and when smiling [10]. Long faces are frequently associated with an excessive anterior display (Fig. 2.10).

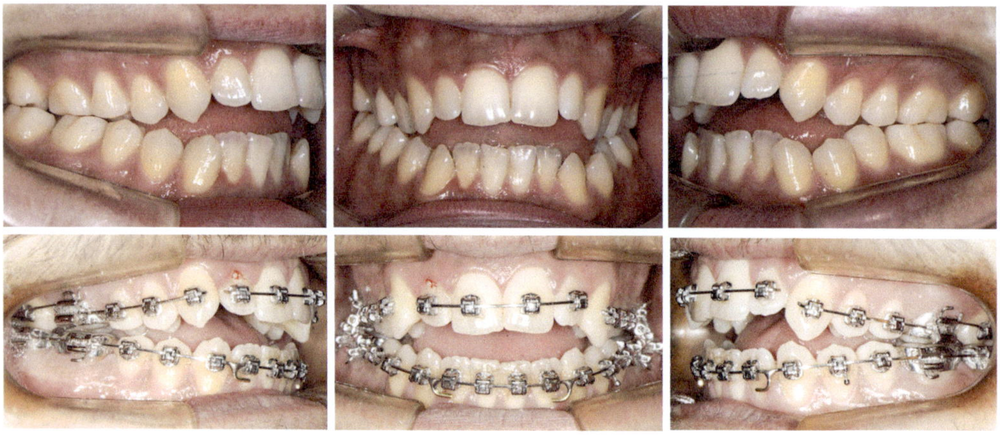

Fig. 2.9 Segmental orthodontic preparation of the upper arch allows for surgical correction of the curve of Spee through maxillary segmental surgery

Fig. 2.10 Gummy smile secondary to vertical maxillary excess is corrected with maxillary impaction

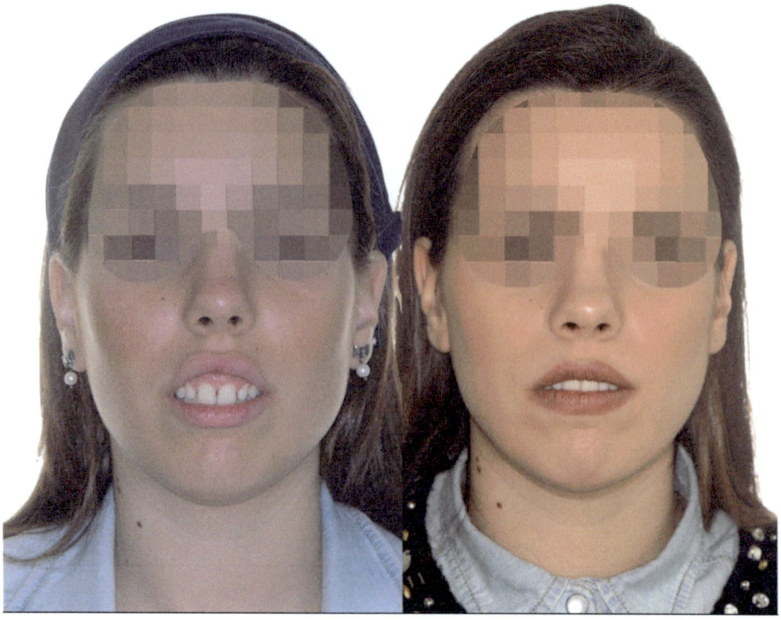

In any case, it is very important to take into consideration the fact that forward repositioning and/or counterclockwise rotation of the maxilla may have an impact on the amount of incisal display. This means that vertical changes measured intraoperatively with the caliper should not be accepted as absolute when a simultaneous advancement and/or counterclockwise rotation of the maxilla takes place. Instead, clinical intraoperative judgment must accompany vertical fine-tuning, and it should be related to lip reaction.

2.3 Labiomental Fold

The labiomental fold is usually absent in long faces. There are two possible causes, alone or combined. First, lack of torque in the lower incisors (the incisor–mandibular plane angle (IMPA) should be orthodontically placed at approximately 90° in relation to the mandibular plane) [4] (Fig. 2.11). Second, lack of chin projection, typically associated with posteriorly rotated mandibles, and which will require an advancement genioplasty (Fig. 2.12).

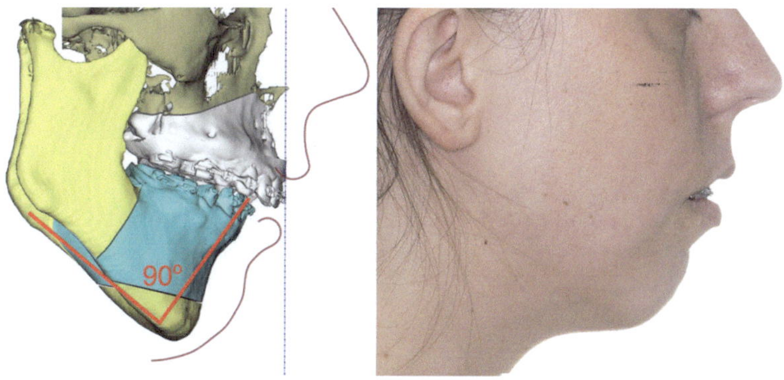

Fig. 2.11 The labiomental sulcus can be defined by adequate torque in the lower incisors and/or adequate chin projection

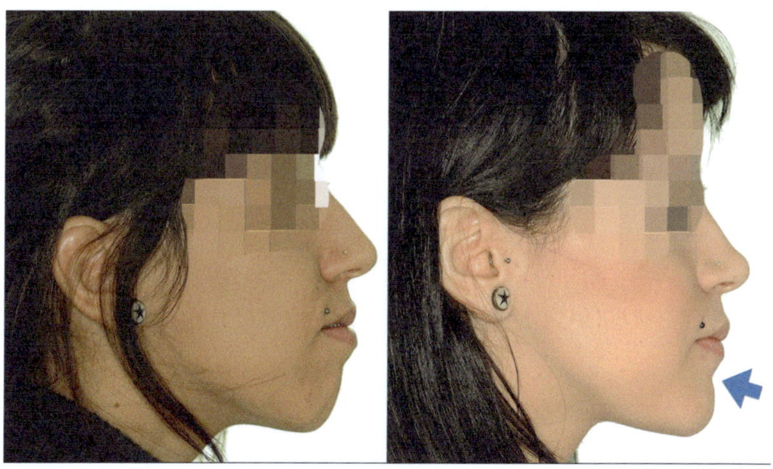

Fig. 2.12 The "long face impression" is enhanced when jawline definition is absent and disappears when it is recovered

A lack of mandibular/chin definition in the frontal view further enhances the "long face impression." In a way, it is as if we were unable to identify "the end of the face." Achievement of an adequate projection of the mandible, usually via counterclockwise rotation, typically provokes this "end of the face" effect, which visually eliminates the "long face impression" (Fig. 2.13).

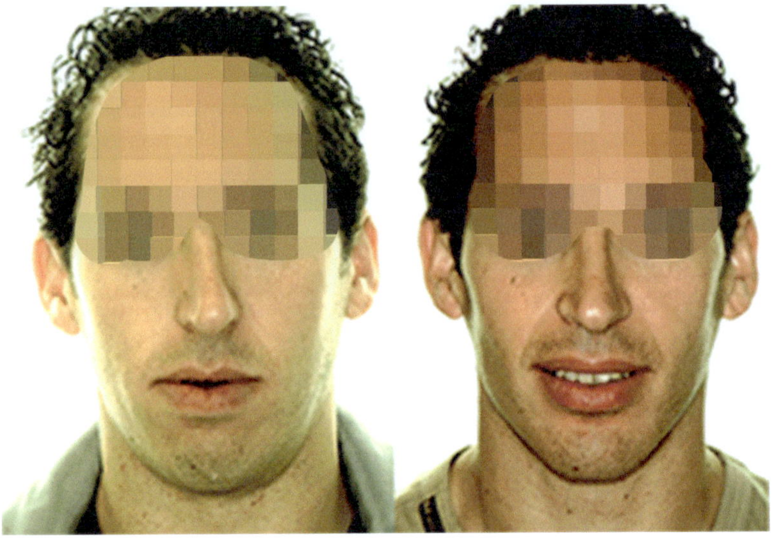

Fig. 2.13 "Long face appearance" is associated with a lack of definition of the "end of the face." Pushing the face forward improves this definition

2.4 Key Points

- Vertical evaluation of the face relies on perception rather than on measurements. The "impression of short or long" is what matters.
- There are four components causing vertical problems: maxillary height, chin height, bite, and transverse dimension of the face.
- Short faces need lengthening. Clockwise maxillomandibular rotation and maxillary downgrafting are the typical movements associated to correction.
- Long faces often do not need shortening but rather the redistribution of components. In the case of shortening of a long face, compensation should be achieved by anterior projection.
- Gummy smile must be carefully analyzed to determine which of the three causes (vertical maxillary excess, lip hypermobility, or altered passive eruption) are implicated.
- The labiomental fold is often absent in long faces because of a lack of incisor torque and/or a receded chin.

References

1. Hernández-Alfaro F, Rozencweig G. Syndrome d'hyperdivergence faciale. [The long face syndrome]. L'Orthodontie Française: Orthod Fr. 2016;87:479–489.
2. Hernández-Alfaro F, Vivas-Castillo J, de Oliveira, Rogerio B, Haas Junior OL, Giralt-Hernando M, Valls-Ontañón A. Barcelona line. A multicenter validation study of a facial projection reference in orthognathic surgery. Br J Oral Maxillofac Surg [Internet] 2022. Available from: https://www.sciencedirect.com/science/article/pii/S0266435622002819.
3. Prittinen JR. Orthodontic diagnosis of long face syndrome. Gen Dent. 1996;44(4):348–51.
4. Prittinen JR. Orthodontic management of long face syndrome. Gen Dent. 1997;45(6):568–72.
5. Haas Junior OL, Guijarro-Martínez R, de Sousa Gil AP, da Silva Meirelles L, de Oliveira RB, Hernández-Alfaro F. Stability and surgical complications in segmental Le Fort I osteotomy: a systematic review [Internet]. Int J Oral Maxillofac Surg Elsevier. 2017;46:1071–87. [cited 2017 Jul 2]. Available from: http://www.ncbi.nlm.nih.gov/pubmed/28601432.
6. Zardawi FM, Gul SS, Fatih MT, Hama BJ. Surgical procedures reducing excessive gingival display in gummy smile patients with various etiologic backgrounds. Clin Adv Periodontics. United States. 2020;10:130–4.
7. Younespour S, Yaghobee S, Aslroosta H, Moslemi N, Pourheydar E, Ghafary ES. Effectiveness of different modalities of lip repositioning surgery for management of patients complaining of excessive gingival display: a systematic review and meta-analysis. Biomed Res Int. 2021;2021:9476013.
8. Dym H, Pierre R 2nd. Diagnosis and treatment approaches to a "gummy smile". Dent Clin N Am. 2020;64(2):341–9.
9. Duruel O, Ataman-Duruel ET, Tözüm TF, Berker E. Ideal dose and injection site for gummy smile treatment with botulinum toxin-a: a systematic review and introduction of a case study. Int J Periodontics Restorative Dent. 2019;39(4):e167–73.
10. Bastidas JA. Surgical correction of the "gummy smile". Oral Maxillofac Surg Clin North Am [Internet]. 2021;33(2):197–209. https://doi.org/10.1016/j.coms.2021.01.005.

3 The Short Face

Federico Hernández-Alfaro

3.1 How Do I Diagnose a Vertical Problem?

Vertical analysis is an essential aspect of aesthetic facial diagnosis and planning [1, 2]. Classical cephalometric analyses have proposed a number of methods to vertically diagnose the face (Fig. 3.1) [3–6]. All of them are based either on numbers or on proportions between different thirds of the face. The most widely accepted norm, coming from the Renaissance masters, is that all three facial thirds should be equal [7].

My personal approach is an aesthetic one and is based on the "impression" of facial length rather than on "measurements" of the facial thirds [8]. Hence, I will define a face as being short, normal, or long, based on my impression [2] (Fig. 3.2).

This approach might seem too naive or subjective, but it is not. Over the last years, in my university seminars and congress lectures worldwide, I have had the opportunity to see that there is a high level of agreement when it comes to subjectively evaluating a face in the vertical dimension, classifying it as normal, short, or long [9].

Looking at all the faces in Fig. 3.3, most readers will agree that they "impress" us as being "short faces." However, if we measure them and apply the classical equal-third cephalometric concept, we will find that they are not. Hence, at this point, we need to agree that it is the first impression, more than a numerical analysis, that prevails when describing a vertical face imbalance [2]. However, this first decision does not say much regarding the cause of and/or solution to the problem. So, what is next?

F. Hernández-Alfaro (✉)
Department of Oral and Maxillofacial Surgery, International University of Catalonia, Barcelona, Spain
e-mail: h.alfaro@uic.es

F. Hernández-Alfaro, A. Valls Ontañón (eds.), *Orthofacial Surgery*,
https://doi.org/10.1007/978-3-031-76185-0_3

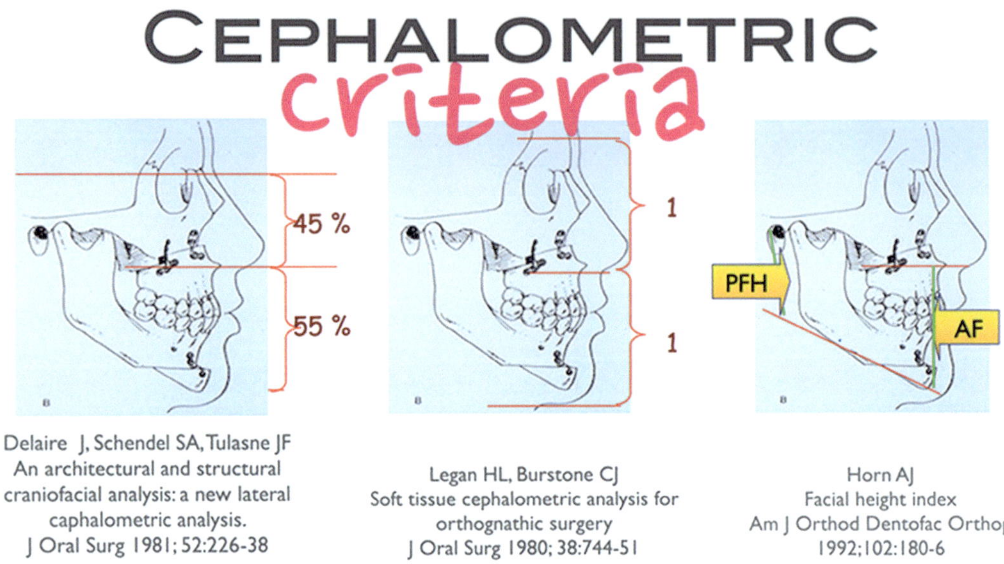

Fig. 3.1 Classical cephalometric analyses have proposed a number of methods to vertically diagnose the face

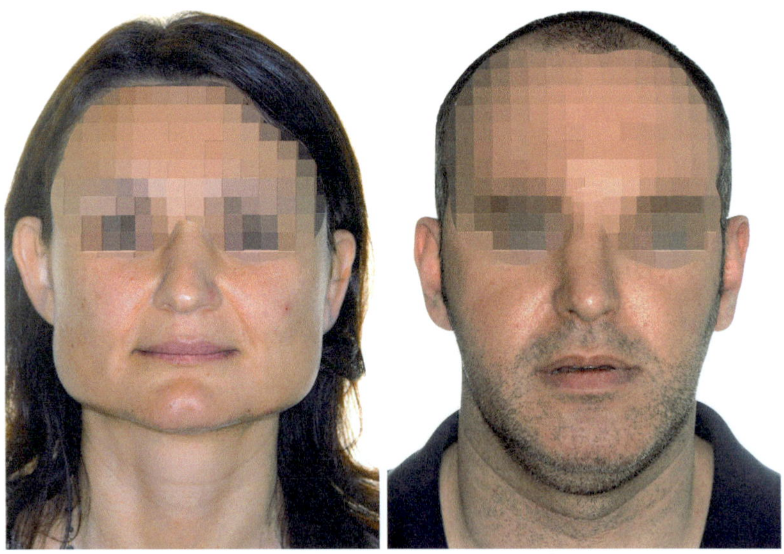

Fig. 3.2 These two faces have equal facial thirds. However, the one on the left "impresses" us as being short and the one on the right as being long

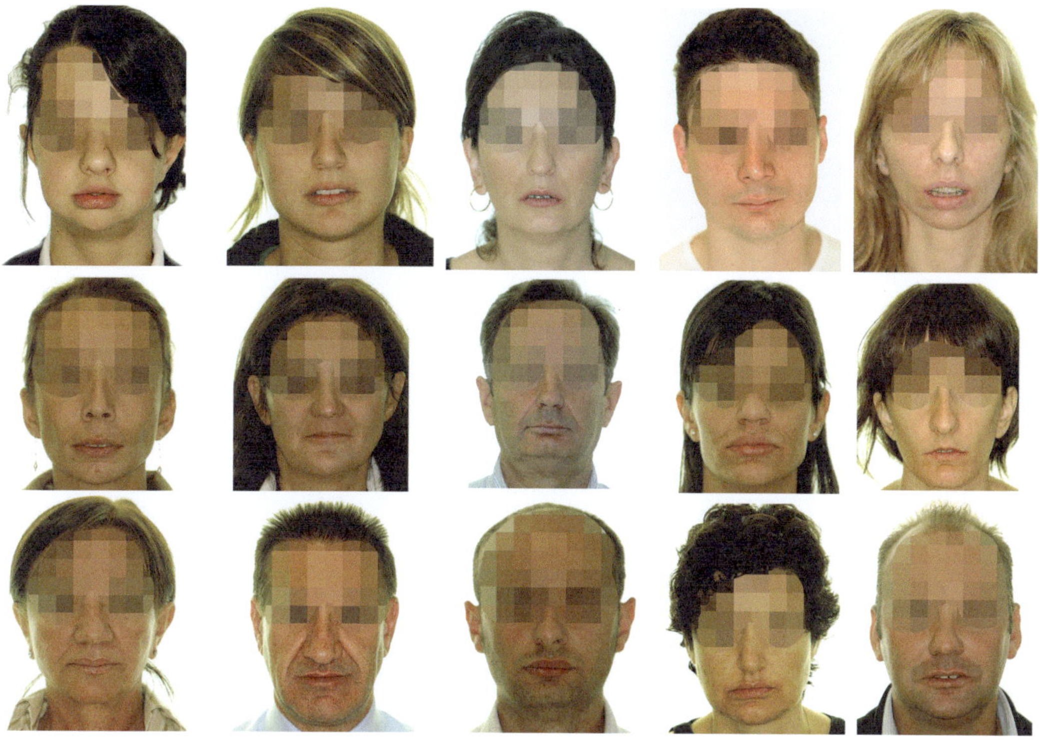

Fig. 3.3 All these faces "impress" us as being short

3.2 Which Are the Components of a Vertical Problem?

Once we have decided that a particular face is short or long, we need to analyze why.

There are four components which—alone or combined—can give the impression of a short or a long face [8], namely.

Vertical dimension of the maxilla: A vertically excessive or deficient maxilla may contribute to a long or short facial appearance (Fig. 3.4).

Vertical dimension of the anterior mandible: Specifically, a long or short chin also influences our vertical perception of the face (Fig. 3.5).

Occlusion: An overbite shortens the face and an open bite lengthens it (Fig. 3.6).

Facial width: A face too large in the transverse dimension contributes to the impression of a short face. The opposite is true for a long face (Fig. 3.7).

Thus, when evaluating a short or long face, we need to know which of these four components are present, and this will largely determine the treatment plan.

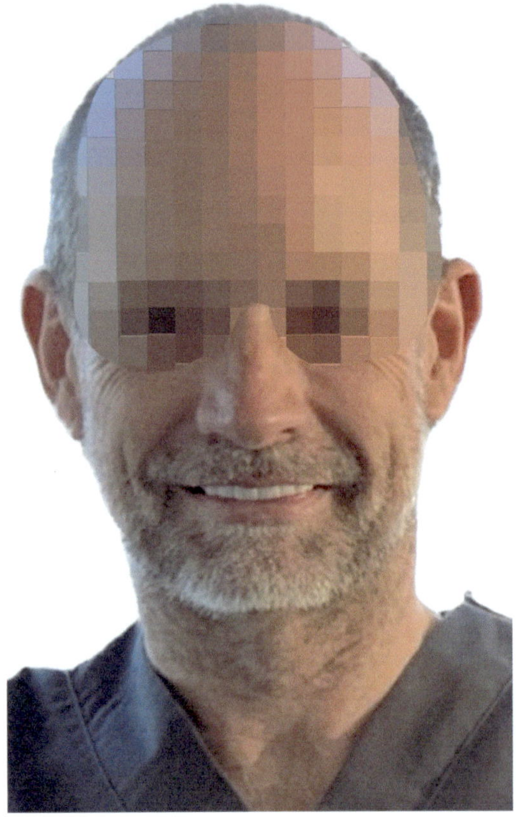

Fig. 3.4 Short face secondary to a vertically short maxilla

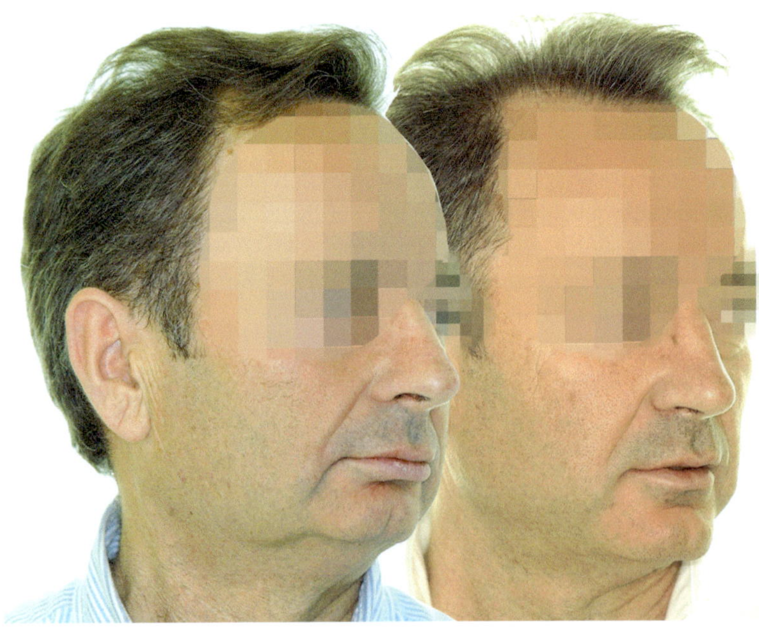

Fig. 3.5 Short face secondary to a vertically short chin

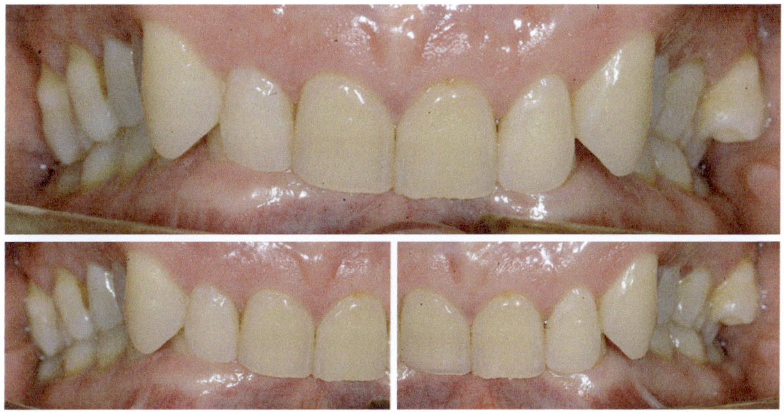

Fig. 3.6 Overbite provokes shortening of the face

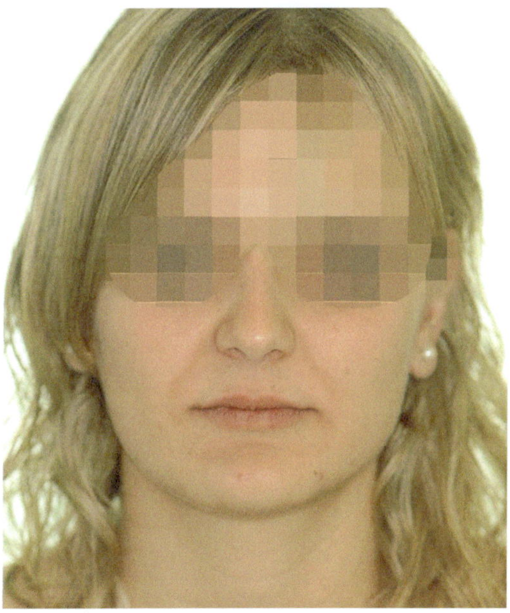

Fig. 3.7. A "wide" face contributes to a short face "appearance"

3.3 Short Face Syndrome

Easily recognized, short faces can be caused by a number of forms of maxillomandibular malpositioning. However, most of them are divided in two very frequent—almost syndromic—groups, depending on the Angle classification of occlusion and the anteroposterior skeletal problem involved [10].

3.3.1 Short Face Low Occlusal Plane

This is the most prevalent presentation among the short faces and is characterized by distinctive facial traits. These patients are easily recognized and typically have a squared and angled face with strong gonial angles, a prominent chin, and overbite.

Based on the occlusion class, we can distinguish the following presentations:

Class II patients: Most of them have a hypoplastic maxilla vertically and anteroposteriorly. The mandible is usually very small, yielding a class II occlusion and overbite.

The typical traits in this group are: *squared face, reduced incisal exposure, deep chin–lip sulcus, excess perimandibular soft tissues, and premature facial aging* (Fig. 3.5).

The management strategy in this situation (in the absence of maxillary problems) consists of mandibular advancement. At our institute, mandibular advancement is performed under local anesthesia and sedation, as published elsewhere [11] and described in Chap. 11 (Fig. 3.8a and b).

Often, however, a small mandible is accompanied by a deficient maxilla. In this scenario, maxillomandibular advancement is necessary, together with clockwise rotation and genioplasty (Fig. 3.9a and b).

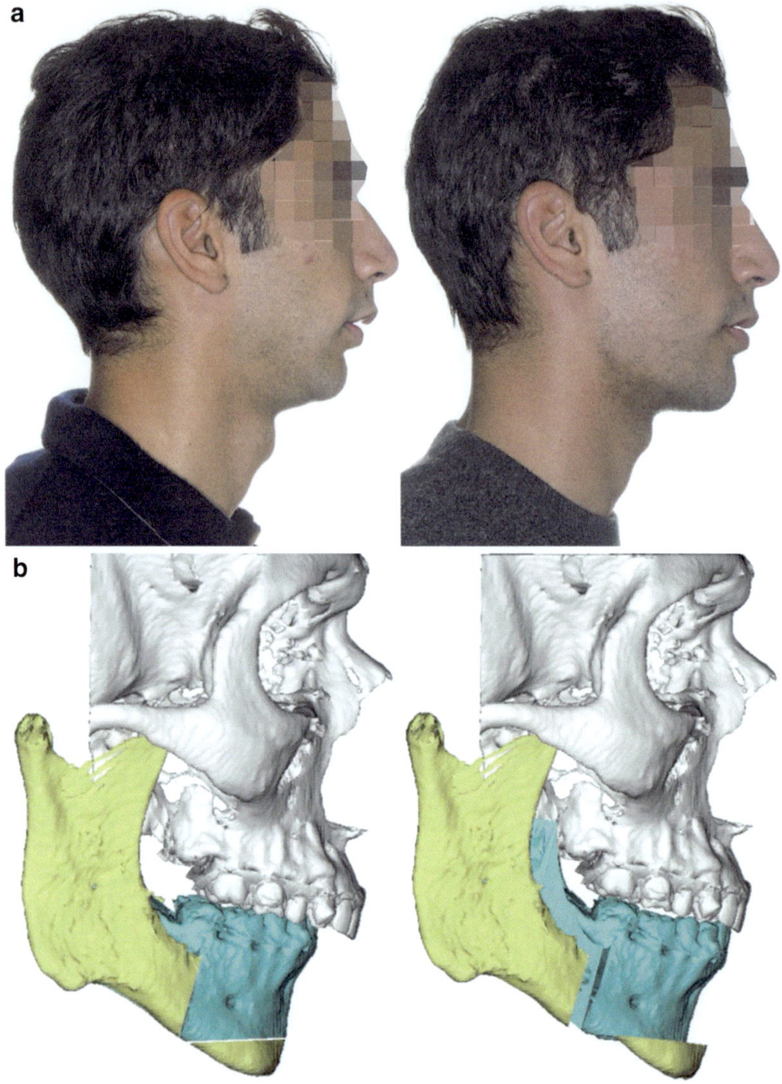

Fig. 3.8 (**a** and **b**) Mandibular advancement to manage a short face and class II patient

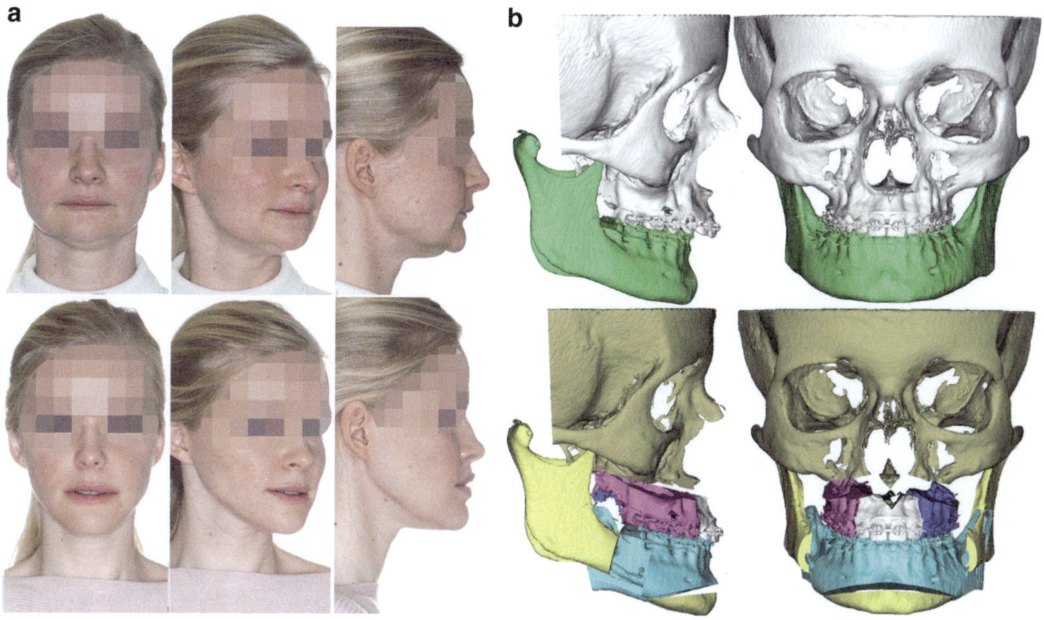

Fig. 3.9 (**a** and **b**) Short face with a low occlusal plane managed through maxillomandibular advancement with clockwise rotation, downgrafting, and "hinge" genioplasty

Class III patients: The typical traits in this case are: *squared face, absent incisal exposure, reduced nasolabial fold, excess middle-third soft tissues, lack of nasal support, and premature facial aging.*

In general terms, the main cause of this situation is a deficient maxilla, both vertically and anteroposteriorly, yielding a class III occlusion and reverse overbite. The solution in the absence of mandibular problems consists of maxillary downgrafting and/or advancement (Fig. 3.10).

3.3.2 Short Face High Occlusal Plane

This is a much less prevalent situation that is usually associated with maxillomandibular retrusion and class II occlusion. These faces are not often "cephalometrically" short but present traits associated with the "short face appearance," such as a lack of incisal exposure and soft tissue sagging. Management usually consists of maxillomandibular advancement plus counterclockwise rotation (Fig. 3.11a–c).

A common problem to be noted in all short faces, regardless of the skeletal cause or occlusion class, is the lack of soft-tissue support and thus premature facial aging. Hence, in any case, facial elongation and expansion should be a primary goal in the management of all short faces.

In the majority of "short face" cases, there is involvement of both the maxilla and the mandible, requiring bimaxillary surgery [12, 13]. In my experience, most short faces present with bimaxillary retrusion and need bimaxillary advancement, combined in most cases with the clockwise rotation of the occlusal plane (Fig. 3.12a and b).

As discussed in Chap. 9, rotational movements of the bimaxillary complex allow us to independently project the paranasal areas and chin (pogonion). Usually, short face patients have a pronounced chin (even with a short mandible) and a lack of support in the paranasal areas. Because of this, "clockwise" is the most common rotational movement associated with these cases. However, there are a few exceptions to this general rule, namely short face patients with posterior divergence, more specifically, patients with a short face and a small mandible and chin (Fig. 3.13a and b).

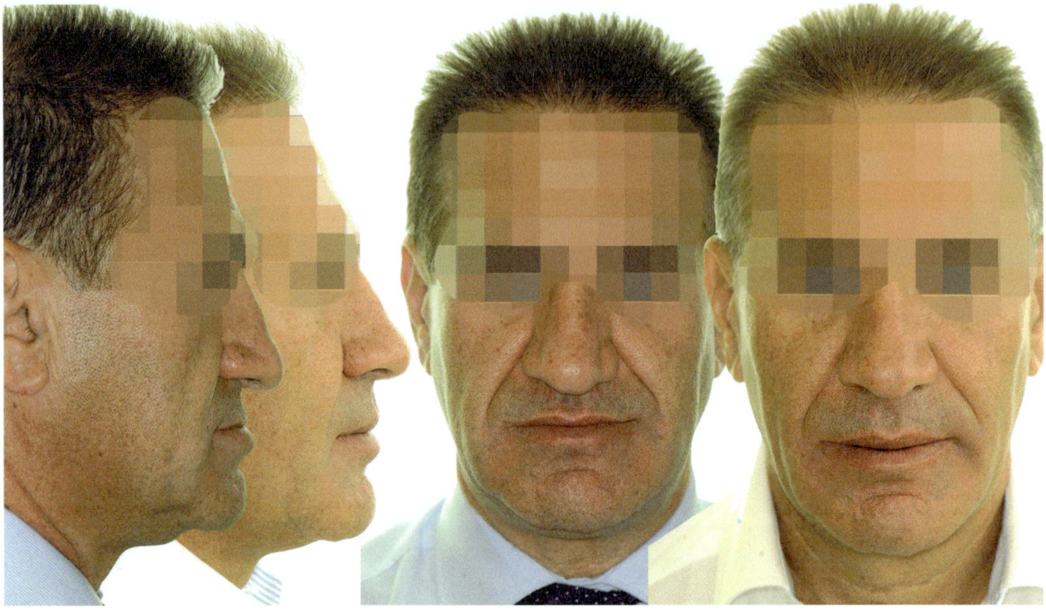

Fig. 3.10 Class III occlusion associated with a short maxilla, both horizontal and vertical, managed through maxillary advancement and downgrafting

Thus, the general therapeutic goals in the management of "short face" patients could be summarized as follows:

1. *Lengthening of the face.*
2. *Achieving class I occlusion and an adequate overbite.*
3. *Correct incisal exposure.*
4. *Induction of anterior projection of the face and increased soft-tissue support (see Chap. 2).*
5. *Affording natural support to the nose.*
6. *Normalization of the inferior labiomental fold.*

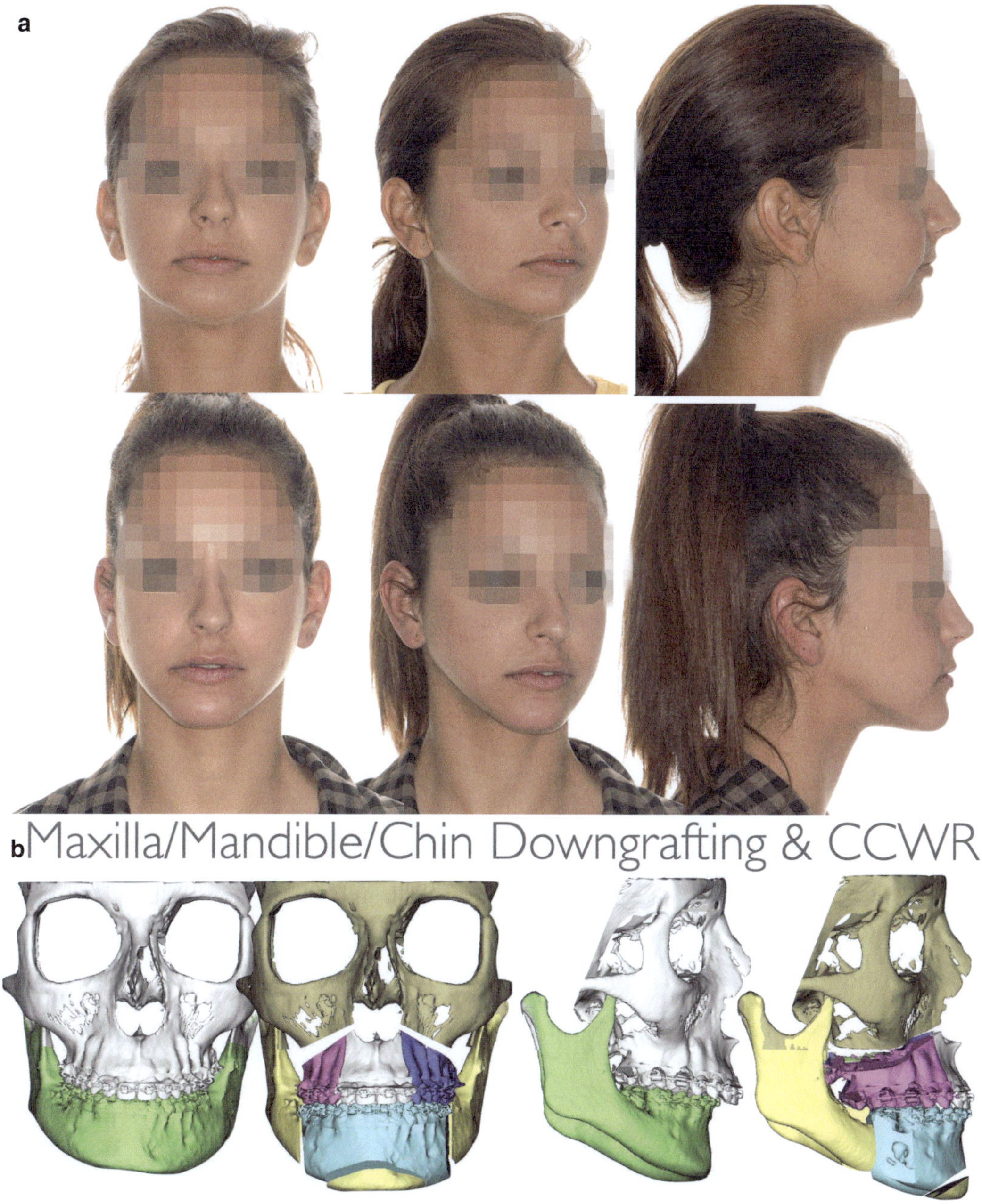

Fig. 3.11 (**a**–**c**) Short face with a high occlusal plane managed through maxillomandibular advancement with counterclockwise rotation and hinge genioplasty

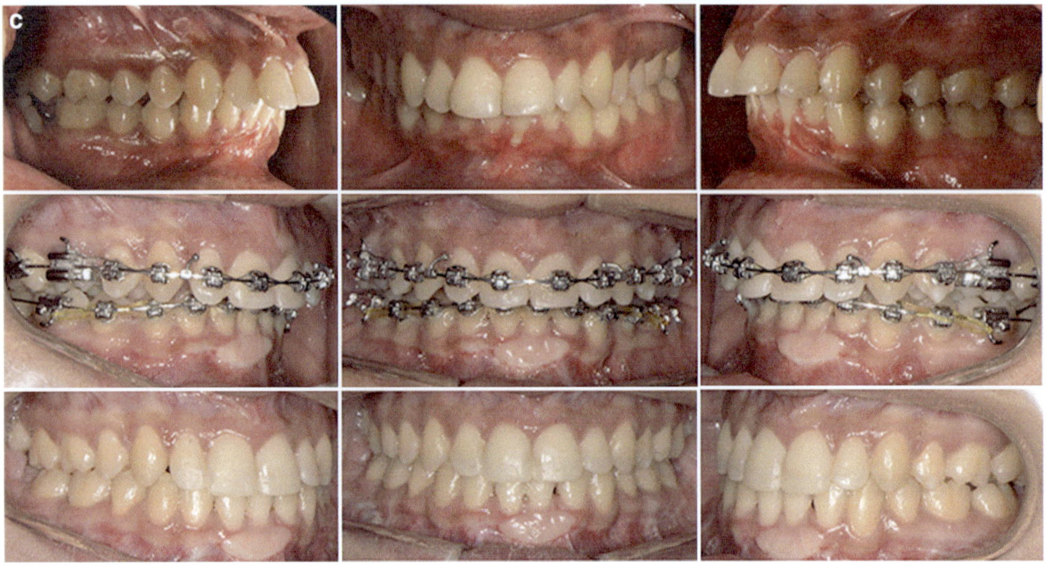

Fig. 3.11 (continued)

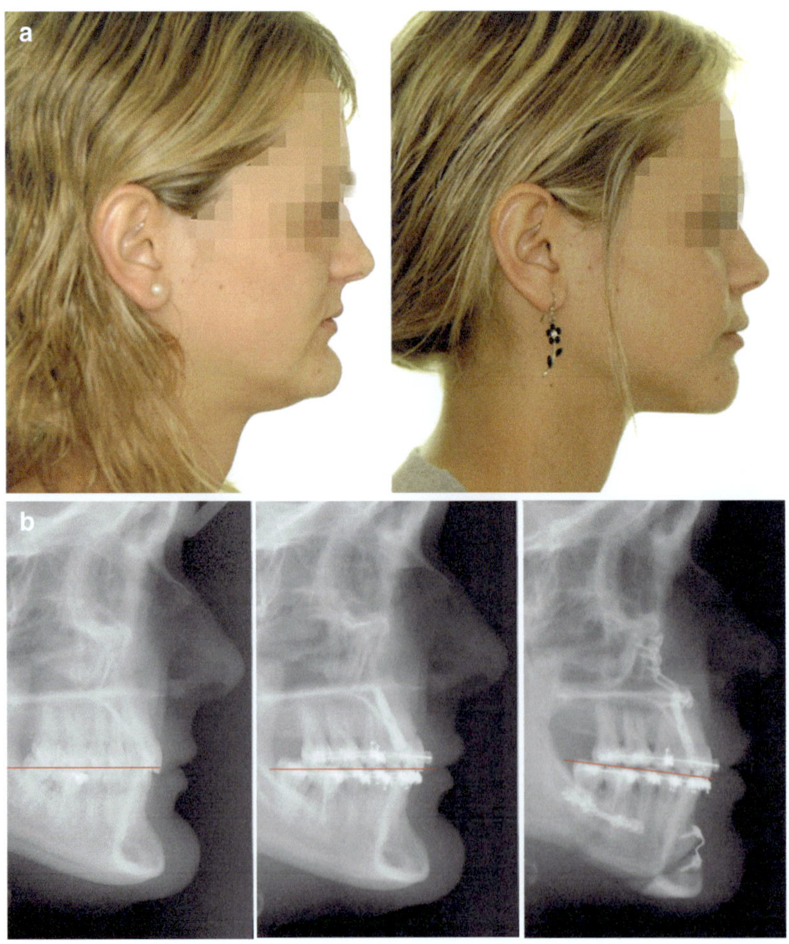

Fig. 3.12 (**a** and **b**) Short face with a low occlusal plane managed through maxillomandibular advancement with clockwise rotation and "hinge" genioplasty

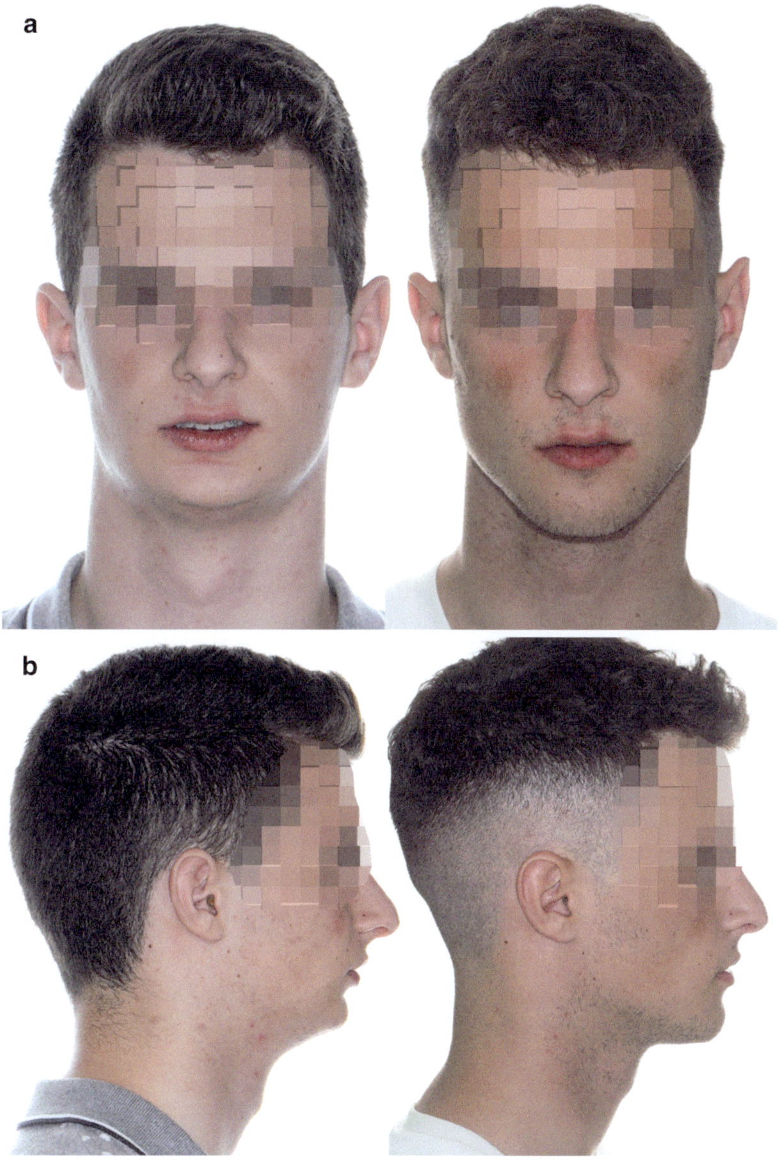

Fig. 3.13 (**a** and **b**) Short face with a high occlusal plane managed through maxillomandibular advancement with counterclockwise rotation, downgrafting, and hinge genioplasty

3.4 Face Lengthening

This can be achieved by downgrafting the maxilla and/or downgrafting the chin (usually with a simultaneous clockwise rotation).

Differential anterior–posterior maxillary downgrafting is needed when rotational movements of the maxillary complex are planned. Clockwise rotation will imply more descent and grafting in the anterior maxilla and the opposite with counterclockwise rotation.

3.5 Incisal Exposure

In order to achieve these goals, most "short face" cases need bimaxillary surgery. Lengthening of the facial skeleton typically induces distraction of the facial mask, more specifically, of the facial muscles. This may entail a greater tendency to relapse, which should be overcome by adequate bone fixation and bone grafting.

A key point in the correction of the short face is to determine the adequate vertical position of the upper incisor (incisor display). Presurgical clinical evaluation allows us to measure the relative position of the upper incisor in relation to the upper lip at rest and when smiling [1]. Theoretically, by measuring this relation, one should be able to determine the amount of maxillary downgrafting needed to normalize the incisor display. However, the fact that most maxillary downgrafting procedures are accompanied by maxillary advancements systematically distorts this preplanned relationship. Hence, in my experience, presurgical measurements and plans should be fine-tuned intraoperatively once the reaction of the lip and paranasal soft tissues to maxillary displacement has been evaluated. This is one of the reasons why I do not use "fully" customized preformed fixation plates [14]. They simply do not allow me to perform this intrasurgical vertical adjustment which, in my experience, is necessary in nearly all cases.

3.6 Labiomental Fold

A deep labiomental fold is arguably one of the main negative traits associated to a class II—short face syndrome. This may be caused by three nonexclusive causes:

1. *Lower lip eversion because of the premature contact with the upper incisors.*
2. *Excessive torque in the lower incisors provoking excessive lower lip projection.*
3. *Excessive chin projection.*

In conclusion, when analyzing and planning "short face" correction, it is of utmost importance to determine which of the previous causes are present and plan for their correction. In this line, the aforementioned scenarios could be managed as follows:

Cause 1 is solved when *mandibular advancement* corrects the class II occlusion and the lower lip no longer touches the upper incisors (Fig. 3.14).

Cause 2 needs to be addressed *orthodontically*, either by stripping, extractions, or distalization with posterior transmucosal attachment devices (TADs).

Cause 3 is managed through a *genioplasty*. I try to avoid setback genioplasties as much as possible, since they tend to cause soft-tissue sagging. Instead, my preference is to perform a "*hinge*" genioplasty which—through clockwise rotation—allows the simultaneous reduction of chin projection and vertical augmentation (Fig. 3.15a and b).

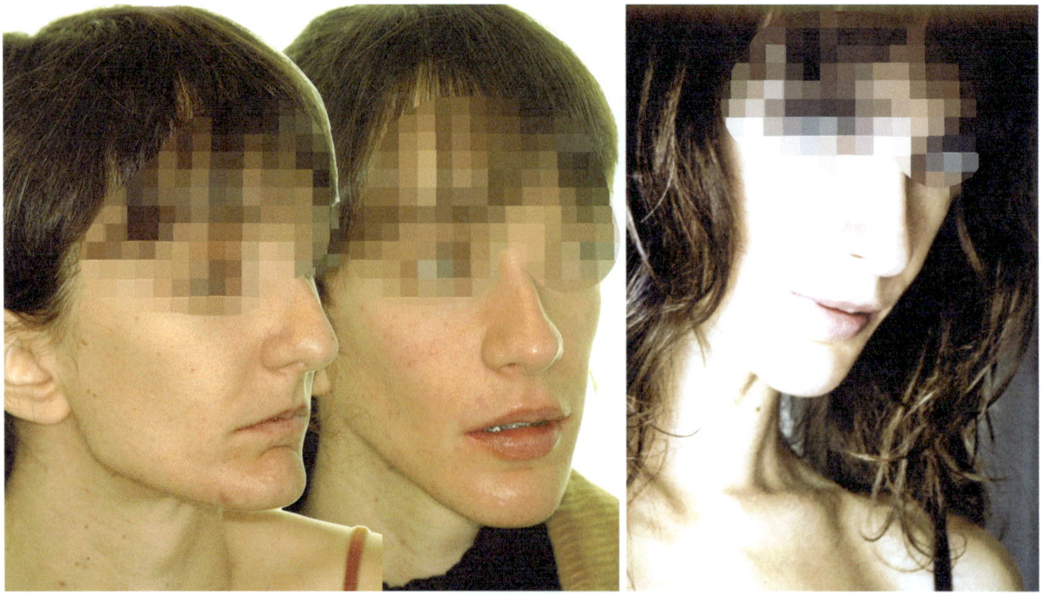

Fig. 3.14 Advancement of the mandible in a short face with class II occlusion contributes to eliminate lower lip eversion

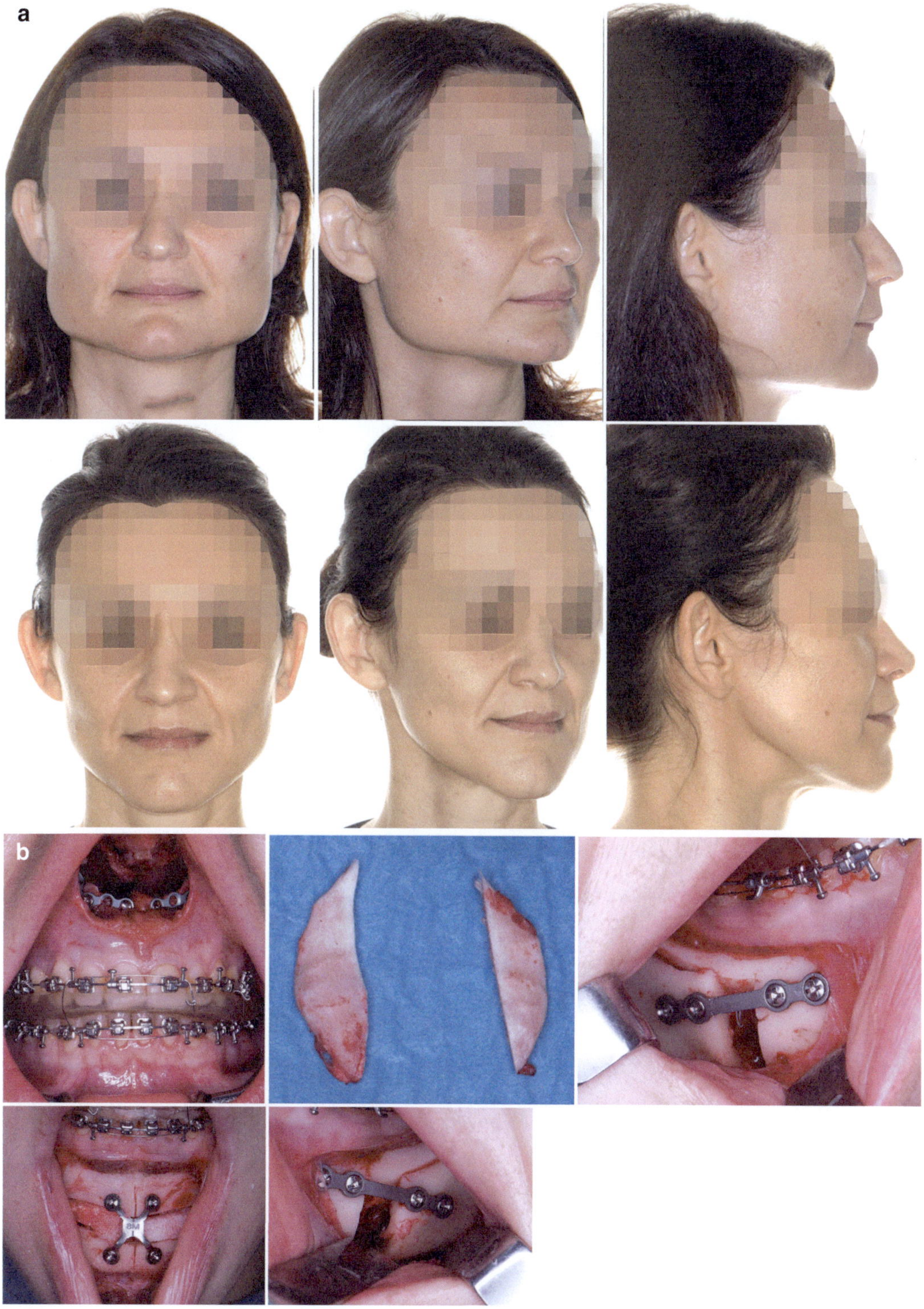

Fig. 3.15 Short face managed through maxillomandibular advancement, clockwise rotation, reduction of mandibular genial angles, and hinge genioplasty

3.7 Key Points

- *Vertical analysis of the face is more about "impressions" than about measurements.*
- *The impression of a short face should be followed by an analysis of the underlying cause, establishing which of the four vertical components of the face are causing this impression, namely, maxillary height, chin height, bite, and face width.*
- *The typical short face is accompanied by a low occlusal plane and needs clockwise rotation as part of the treatment plan.*
- *A lack of upper incisor exposure is also a common short face trait and is corrected by maxillary anterior downgrafting.*
- *A deep labiomental fold is due to a short and overprojected chin and/or excessive lower incisor torque.*

References

1. Hernández-Alfaro F. Upper incisor to Soft Tissue Plane (UI-STP): a new reference for diagnosis and planning in dentofacial deformities. Med Oral Patol Oral Cir Bucal. 2010;15(5):8–10.
2. Hernández-Alfaro F, Vivas-Castillo J, de Oliveira, RB, Haas Junior OL, Giralt-Hernando M, Valls-Ontañón A. Barcelona line. A multicenter validation study of a facial projection reference in orthognathic surgery. Br J Oral Maxillofac Surg [Internet]. 2022; Available from: https://www.sciencedirect.com/science/article/pii/S0266435622002819.
3. Delaire J, Schendel SA, Tulasne JF. An architectural and structural craniofacial analysis: a new lateral cephalometric analysis. Oral Surg Oral Med Oral Pathol. 1981;52(3):226–38.
4. Legan HL, Burstone CJ. Soft tissue cephalometric analysis for orthognathic surgery. J Oral Surg. 1980;38(10):744–51.
5. Horn AJ. Facial height index. Am J Orthod Dentofacial Orthop. 1992;102(2):180–6.
6. Shindoi JM, Matsumoto Y, Sato Y, Ono T, Harada K. Soft tissue cephalometric norms for orthognathic and cosmetic surgery. J Oral Maxillofac Surg. 2013;71(1):e24–30.
7. Pancherz H, Knapp V, Erbe C, Heiss AM. Divine proportions in attractive and nonattractive faces. World J Orthod. 2010;11(1):27–36.
8. Hernández-alfaro F, Rozencweig G. Syndrome d'hyperdivergence faciale. 2016;87:479–89.
9. Freihofer HP. Surgical treatment of the short face syndrome. J Oral Surg [Internet]. 1981;39(11):907–11. Available from: http://europepmc.org/abstract/MED/6945418.
10. Katz MI. Angle classification revisited 2: a modified Angle classification. Am J Orthod Dentofac Orthop. 1992 Sep;102(3):277–84.
11. Raffaini M, Hernandez Alfaro F, Ghilardi R, Garcia LA. The sagittal mandibular osteotomy under local anesthesia and intravenous sedation: four years of multicenter experience. Int J Adult Orthodon Orthognath Surg. 2002;17(4):267–71.
12. Posnick JC, Ogunsanya O, Singh N, Kinard BE. Short face dentofacial deformities: changes in social perceptions, facial esthetics, and occlusion after bimaxillary and chin orthognathic correction. J Craniofac Surg. 2020;31(3):632–36.
13. Foletti J-M, Antonarakis GS, Vanden Eynden X, Courvoisier DS, Scolozzi P. Is preoperative maintenance of the curve of Spee associated with an increase of facial height in class II short face orthognathic patients? A never answered dogmatic question. J Oral Maxillofac Surg. 2018;76(12):2638–45.
14. Claus JDP, Almeida MS, Hernandez-Alfaro F. In-house hybrid technique for customization of guides and miniplates in orthognathic surgery. J Craniofac Surg. 2020;31(4):1122–4.

4 Transverse Problems

Federico Hernández-Alfaro

4.1 Introduction

Transverse skeletal maxillomandibular discrepancy can be defined as a difference (measured at the posterior alveolar level) of over 4 mm (Fig. 4.1). In growing patients, most transverse discrepancies can be resolved with orthopedic treatment through rapid palatal expansion. This allows for the opening of an incompletely fused midpalatal suture and through bone distraction principles eventually results in a wider maxilla [1–4].

Recently, with the incorporation of the miniscrew-assisted rapid palatal expansion (MARPE) technique, a significant proportion of young adults (under age 25) can be managed nonsurgically with bone-borne devices.

In grown patients, all cranial sutures are fused. Hence, some sort of surgical aid is usually needed in order to allow reopening of the midpalatal suture, simultaneously releasing both the piriform and malar buttresses [5, 6].

F. Hernández-Alfaro (✉)
Department of Oral and Maxillofacial Surgery, International University of Catalonia, Barcelona, Spain
e-mail: h.alfaro@uic.es

F. Hernández-Alfaro, A. Valls Ontañón (eds.), *Orthofacial Surgery*,
https://doi.org/10.1007/978-3-031-76185-0_4

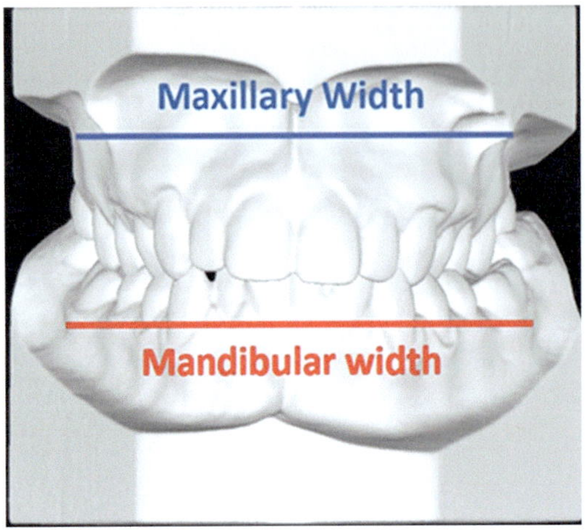

Fig. 4.1 Transverse width/discrepancy needs to be measured at the bone level

We have designed a specific protocol in order to decide which surgical procedure is needed in each clinical scenario [7].

4.2 Maxilla Segmentation

In cases in which maxillary surgery is indicated for some reason (vertical and anteroposterior), and the transverse discrepancy is less than 7 mm, maxillary expansion is achieved through segmentation [8]. Although described in Chap. 10, the basic steps of this procedure are as follows:

- Minimally invasive Le Fort I [9, 10] according to our technique described in Chap. 10.
- Interdental osteotomies typically between lateral and cuspid with a piezoelectric saw, taking care not to elevate the mucoperiosteal flap beyond the mucogingival junction, in order to avoid periodontal problems. (Fig. 4.2a and b). Occasionally, if the curve of Spee becomes pronounced between cuspids and bicuspids, interdental osteotomies can be performed at this point, provided no increase in intercanine width is necessary. For this last scenario, we have published a technique which allows performing interdental osteotomies at this point while still maintaining our reduced approach [11].
- Longitudinal osteotomies also with the piezoelectric saw are performed on the nasal floor, parallel to the septal crest in the maxillary floor.
- A horizontal-connecting final osteotomy is made behind the nasopalatine duct (Fig. 4.3).
- An "H"-shaped osteotomy is thus defined, yielding four fragments which allow for maxillary expansion (Fig. 4.4).

Release of the four segments is carefully achieved by palatal subperiosteal elevation under the lateral segments. Ideally, the posterior vascular pedicles should be preserved in order to maintain an adequate blood supply to all segments.

Performing two longitudinal osteotomies instead of a single midpalatal one allows us to split the amount of expansion on both sides, reducing the size of the gap on each.

The four segments are then included in the splint, fixing it with wire ligatures around the braces. In cases where no buccal braces are in place (lingual orthodontics, aligners), five

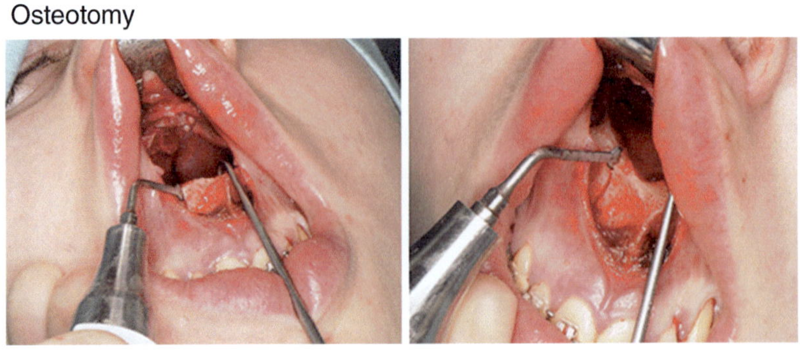

Fig. 4.2 Interdental osteotomies are performed with a piezoelectric saw, avoiding damage to the mucosa and periosteum

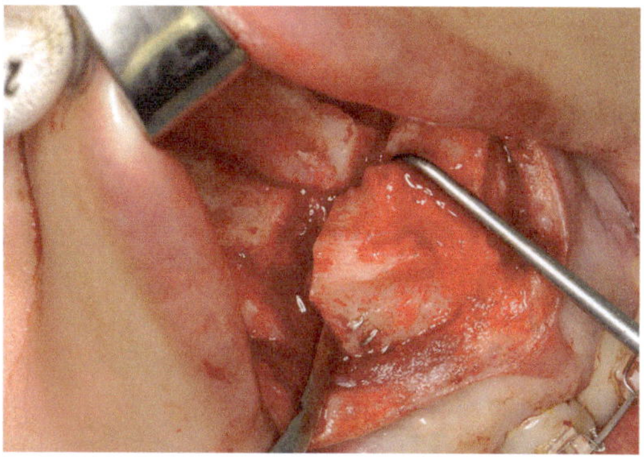

Fig. 4.3 Full mobilization of the four fragments after completing the osteotomies

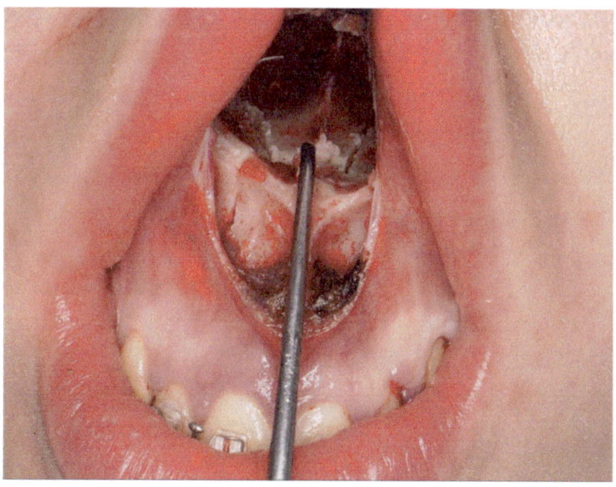

Fig. 4.4 Four-piece segmental osteotomies through the same reduced approach

mini-screws are placed in the maxillary segments, and the splint is wired to them.

At the end of the procedure, we remove the final CAD/CAM splint and place a palatal removable plate with an expansion screw. This allows for transverse stability and, if needed, further expansion of the segments.

4.3 SARPE/SAMARPE

This procedure is indicated in skeletally mature patients with an isolated transverse maxillary deficiency and patients who will eventually sustain a regular orthognathic procedure but have a transverse discrepancy in excess of 6 mm that cannot be resolved through segmentation.

Surgically assisted rapid palatal expansion (SARPE) consists of the surgical release of the sites of resistance combined using orthopedic forces. Thanks to the principles of osteogenic distraction, SARPE can widen the upper arch in skeletally mature patients. Several technical approaches have been advocated since the first description by Brown [12], who used a medial palatal osteotomy—the hypothesis being that this area is the most resistant to maxillary expansion. Since then, several authors have proposed different areas of resistance and advocated several combined osteotomies to mobilize them [13, 14]. The areas of resistance have been classified as anterior support (piriform aperture pillars), lateral support (zygomatic buttresses), posterior support (pterygoid junctions), and medial support (midpalatal suture). The reviewed literature evidences no consensus regarding the extent of the necessary osteotomies for SARPE [14, 15].

Most technical descriptions advocate the use of general anesthesia with hospital admission [16]. Bays and Greco [17] proposed local anesthesia plus sedation as an ambulatory procedure but only for cases where pterygomaxillary disjunction is not needed. In such cases, posterior expansion is limited.

Our previously published surgical technique [11, 18, 19] involves the full release of all areas of resistance, namely, midpalatal, piriform, zygomatic, and pterygoid. We always perform this procedure under local anesthesia and sedation on an ambulatory basis.

Patients are instructed to rinse their mouth before the procedure, to be accompanied, and to wear comfortable clothes. Local anesthetic (articaine with epinephrine) plus mild intravenous sedation consisting of midazolam and remifentanil is administered in the operating room at our surgical office. Surgical field isolation is achieved through sterile drapes after scrub decontamination of the face with iodine.

The first step consists of the release of the pterygomaxillary suture with a piezoelectric saw through a transmucosal approach, as published by our group [11, 19].

A 10 mm through-and-through buccal incision over the keratinized mucosa limit is performed with a Colorado needle. The incision runs horizontally to reach the level of the laterals. Periosteal elevation is then performed with a sharp instrument, degloving the maxillary bone from the piriform aperture to the pterygomaxillary junction. The vertical width of the exposed area at the maxilla is sufficient to allow osteotomies to be performed. Subspinal osteotomy is achieved with the piezoelectric saw to preserve a fair number of insertions of the nasal base muscles and reduce postoperative nasal widening. Subperiosteal dissection of the nasal floor and deinsertion of the septal base are achieved with a narrow periosteal elevator. A piezoelectric saw is used to perform the interincisal through-and-through osteotomy. At this point, a reciprocating saw with a 4 cm blade is used to perform the horizontal osteotomies. The nasal periosteum is protected with a spatula, and a Langenbeck retractor with an inverted tip is used to protect the periosteum laterally and posteriorly. Next, lateral osteotomies are completed with a sharp 2 cm osteotome to reach the pterygomaxillary junction [19] (Figs. 4.5 and 4.6).

Pterygomaxillary osteotomies in the classical lateral approach are not performed. Instead, the piezoelectric saw with a long inset is applied transmucosal at the pterygomaxillary junction, progressing from down below superiorly.

The Hyrax (SARPE) or a mini-screw-anchored device (SAMARPE) (Fig. 4.7) is then activated to check the symmetrical and complete expansion of both sides. One millimeter (four expander activations) expansion remains at the time of surgery. Cross-suturing of the muscles, as described in our paper [19, 20], is achieved using 4/0 Vicryl. Interrupted sutures are used in the vertical segment, and running sutures are placed laterally. Patients are discharged after recovery from sedation [20]. Five to seven days after surgery, patients are instructed to have the expander activated [20].

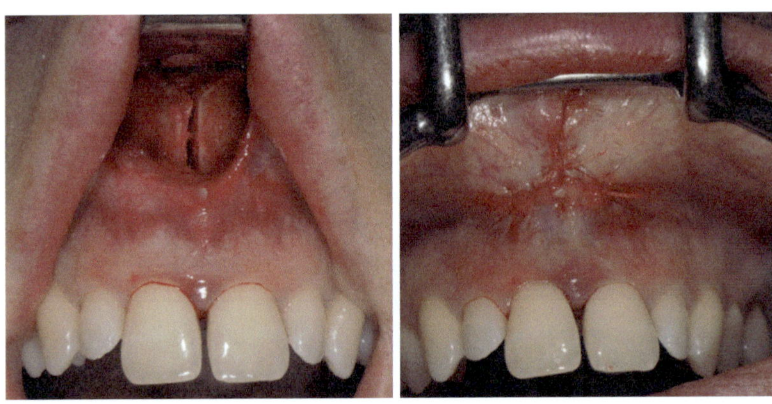

Fig. 4.5 Minimally invasive approach for SARPE

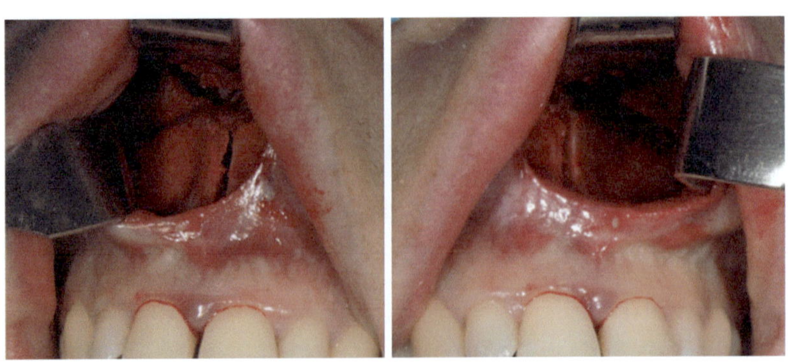

Fig. 4.6 Bilateral horizontal and midline osteotomies

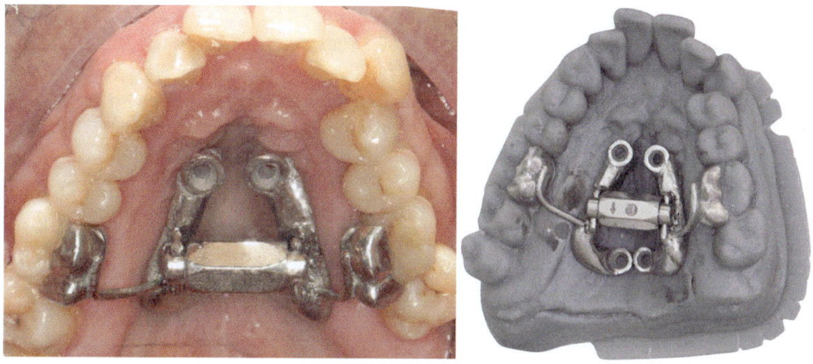

Fig. 4.7 Fully customized bone-borne maxillary expander

4.4 Mandibular Contraction

Contraction of the mandibular arch is another potential solution for transverse discrepancies. It is indicated in our protocol in cases where a class II or III malocclusion is present in need of mandibular surgery with a concomitant transverse discrepancy of less than 7 mm and a three-dimensional (3D) correctly positioned maxilla.

The procedure basically consists of performing a bilateral sagittal osteotomy and simultaneously an additional midline osteotomy. An occlusal splint is essential in order to three-dimensionally position the two resulting segments of the mandible (Fig. 4.8). Then, osteosynthesis is applied in the lateral and midline osteotomies.

Usually, when contracting the arch, a fulcrum appears at the buccal side of the midline osteotomy, generating an anterior gap which needs bone grafting.

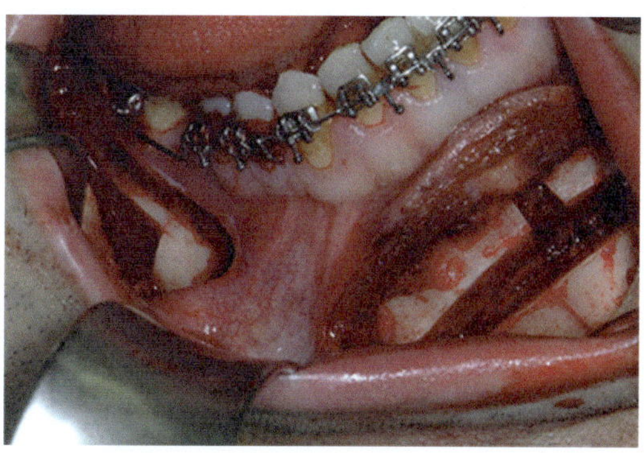

Fig. 4.8 Bilateral sagittal split osteotomy and genioplasty combined with midsymphyseal osteotomy to allow mandibular contraction

4.5 Key Points

- Maxillomandibular transverse discrepancy is a prevalent condition.
- Nonsurgical MARPE is worth trying in patients under age 25.
- SARPE or SAMARPE is the indicated procedure in adult patients.
- Maxilla segmentation is indicated when the transverse discrepancy is less than 7 mm in the context of maxillary surgery.
- Mandibular contraction is indicated when skeletal class II or III malocclusion is accompanied by less than 7 mm of transverse discrepancy and a correctly positioned maxilla.

References

1. Caprioglio A, Castiglioni F, Sambataro S, Giuntini V, Comaglio I, Lorvetti F, et al. Changes in canine inclination after rapid and slow maxillary expansion compared to untreated controls. Orthod Craniofac Res. 2020;23(3):351–6.
2. Sayar G, Kılınç DD. Rapid maxillary expansion outcomes according to midpalatal suture maturation levels. Prog Orthod. 2019;20(1):27.
3. Abdalla Y, Brown L, Sonnesen L. Effects of rapid maxillary expansion on upper airway volume: a three-dimensional cone-beam computed tomography study. Angle Orthod. 2019;89(6):917–23.
4. Di Ventura A, Lanteri V, Farronato G, Gaffuri F, Beretta M, Lanteri C, et al. Three-dimensional evaluation of rapid maxillary expansion anchored to primary molars: direct effects on maxillary arch and spontaneous mandibular response. Eur J Paediatr Dent. 2019;20(1):38–42.
5. Isfeld D, Flores-Mir C, Leon-Salazar V, Lagravère M. Evaluation of a novel palatal suture maturation

classification as assessed by cone-beam computed tomography imaging of a pre- and postexpansion treatment cohort. Angle Orthod. 2019;89(2):252–61.
6. Reyneke JP, Conley RS. Surgical/orthodontic correction of transverse maxillary discrepancies. Oral Maxillofac Surg Clin North Am. 2020;32(1):53–69.
7. Camps-Pereperez I, Guijarro-Martinez R, Peiro-Guijarro MA, Hernandez-Alfaro F. The value of cone beam computed tomography imaging in surgically assisted rapid palatal expansion: a systematic review of the literature. Int J Oral Maxillofac Surg. 2017;46:827.
8. Haas Junior OL, Guijarro-Martínez R, de Sousa Gil AP, da Silva ML, de Oliveira RB, Hernández-Alfaro F. Stability and surgical complications in segmental Le Fort I osteotomy: a systematic review [Internet]. Int J Oral Maxillofac Surg Elsevier. 2017;46:1071–87. [cited 2017 Jul 2]. Available from: http://www.ncbi.nlm.nih.gov/pubmed/28601432.
9. Hernandez-Alfaro F, Guijarro-Martinez R. "Twist technique" for pterygomaxillary dysjunction in minimally invasive Le Fort I osteotomy. J Oral Maxillofac Surg. 2013;71(2):389–92.
10. de Sousa Gil AP, Guijarro-Martínez R, Haas OLJ, Masià-Gridilla J, Valls-Ontañón A, de Oliveira RB, et al. Nasolabial soft tissue effects of segmented and non-segmented Le Fort I osteotomy using a modified alar cinch technique-a cone beam computed tomography evaluation. Int J Oral Maxillofac Surg. 2020;49(7):889–94.
11. Valls-Ontañón A, Hernández-Margarit P, Mazarro-Campos A, Hernández-Alfaro F. Transmucosal posterior segmentation in the context of minimally invasive Le Fort I osteotomy: technical note. J Stomatol Oral Maxillofac Surg France. 2022;123:e82–4.
12. Brown GVI. The surgery of oral and facial diseases and malformations. Londres: Kimpton; 1938. 507 p
13. Bell WH, Epker BN. Surgical-orthodontic expansion of the maxilla. Am J Orthod. 1976;70(5):517–28.
14. Kennedy JW 3rd, Bell WH, Kimbrough OL, James WB. Osteotomy as an adjunct to rapid maxillary expansion. Am J Orthod. 1976;70(2):123–37.
15. Suri L, Taneja P. Surgically assisted rapid palatal expansion: a literature review. Am J Orthod Dentofacial Orthop. 2008;133(2):290–302.
16. Pogrel MA, Kaban LB, Vargervik K, Baumrind S. Surgically assisted rapid maxillary expansion in adults. Int J Adult Orthodon Orthognath Surg. 1992;7(1):37–41.
17. Bays RA, Greco JM. Surgically assisted rapid palatal expansion: an outpatient technique with long-term stability. J Oral Maxillofac Surg. 1992 Feb;50(2):110–5.
18. Hernández Alfaro F, Paternostro Betancourt D, Haas Junior OL, Valls Ontañón A. Customized guide for transmucosal pterygomaxillary disjunction: proof of concept. J Stomatol Oral Maxillofac Surg. 2022;000:3–6.
19. Hernández-Alfaro F, Ghuloom M, Giralt-Hernando M, Lázaro-Abdulkarim A, Valls-Ontañón A. Transmucosal pterygomaxillary disjunction using a piezoelectric device, in the context of the minimally invasive Le Fort I osteotomy protocol. Int J Oral Maxillofac Surg. 2022;52:569.
20. Hernandez-Alfaro F, Mareque Bueno J, Diaz A, Pagés CM. Minimally invasive surgically assisted rapid palatal expansion with limited approach under sedation: a report of 283 consecutive cases. J Oral Maxillofac Surg. 2010;68(9):2154–8.

Facial Asymmetry

5

Federico Hernández-Alfaro,
Orion-Luiz Haas-Junior, and Adaia Valls Ontañón

Complete facial symmetry does not exist in humans. Even the most aesthetic faces present some degree of asymmetry. The single most common causal factor of facial asymmetry is the mandible. Irrespective of the cause, any unilateral disturbance in mandibular growth has an almost immediate impact upon facial harmony in the frontal plane and also in relation to occlusion [1–4].

The younger the patient and/or the longer the period before the diagnosis and treatment of the condition, the greater the asymmetry and involvement of the rest of the facial skeleton will be, particularly the maxilla. Maxillary asymmetry is usually a sequel of mandibular asymmetrical growth and must be treated with dentoalveolar decompensation—orthodontically and/or surgically.

Orthodontic management of asymmetric cases is usually a challenge, since most patients present dental compensations in all three planes of space, apart from the usual dentoalveolar compensations in the anterior maxilla and mandible. Asymmetric cases tend to have posterior transverse (Wilson curve) compensations [5, 6]. Preoperative decompensation of these cases is crucial in order to achieve adequate skeletal repositioning not only in the sagittal but also in the three-dimensional (3D) plane of view—pitch, roll, and yaw (Fig. 5.1a and b).

For diagnosis and management purposes, we will divide this chapter into hypoplastic and hyperplastic conditions.

F. Hernández-Alfaro (✉) · A. Valls Ontañón
Department of Oral and Maxillofacial Surgery, International University of Catalonia, Barcelona, Spain
e-mail: h.alfaro@uic.es; avalls@uic.es

O.-L. Haas-Junior
Department of Oral and Maxillofacial Surgery, Hospital São Lucas – Pontifícia Universidade Católica do Rio Grande do Sul, Porto Alegre, Brazil

Blanc Hospital, Porto Alegre, Brazil

F. Hernández-Alfaro, A. Valls Ontañón (eds.), *Orthofacial Surgery*,
https://doi.org/10.1007/978-3-031-76185-0_5

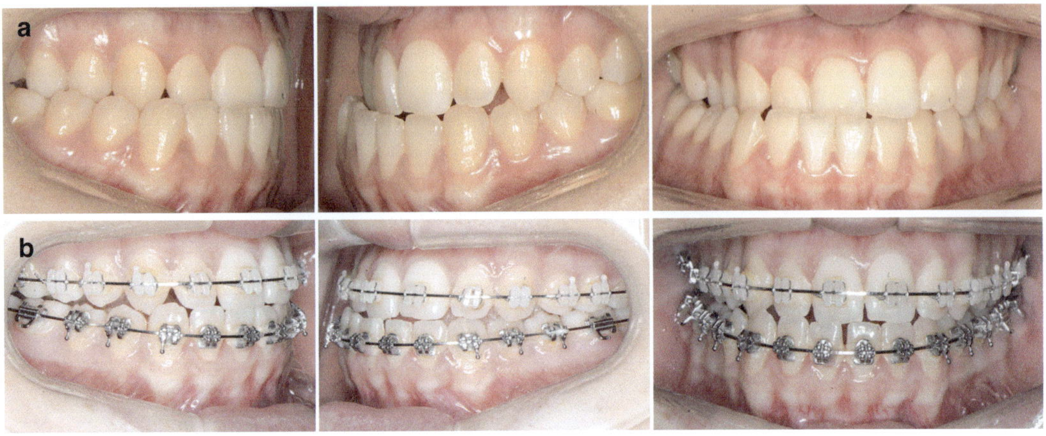

Fig. 5.1 (**a** and **b**) Orthodontic management in complex asymmetries requires full decompensation in all three planes of space.

5.1 Asymmetry Secondary to Unilateral Mandibular Hypoplasia

Mandibular unilateral hypoplasia is most frequently associated to trauma (very often inadvertent) or rheumatic conditions, with underdevelopment of one of the condylar growth centers. When the provoking factor upon the mandible appears during growth, there is usually compensation from the maxilla which typically determines canting of the occlusal plane. The earlier the onset, the more severe the resulting facial asymmetry [7]. Likewise, early onset and late detection/treatment tend to produce functional adaptations of the soft tissues, including the muscles. Hence, the resulting facial asymmetry tends to have both a skeletal and a soft-tissue component.

When this situation is detected during growth, orthopedic management with functional appliances may correct or at least reduce the severity of the problem. If severe, the condition might require osteogenic distraction of the short side of the mandible [8]. In cases of either ankylosis or absence of the condyle, reconstruction with costochondral grafts is often indicated [9].

When the condition is diagnosed in grown patients, our treatment of choice is bimaxillary surgery. If there is concomitant ankylosis or a severe structural anomaly of the condyle, we would simultaneously perform total joint replacement with a fully customized prosthesis (Fig. 5.2a–e).

Apart from an asymmetrically positioned mandible, patients often present with an abnormal morphology, especially at the level of the gonial angles. We have two different strategies to correct this.

First, in mild cases, we perform the original bilateral sagittal split osteotomy (BSSO), as described by Obwegeser, which allows us to lower the mandibular angle at the hypoplastic side (Fig. 5.3a and b).

Second, in more severe cases, our choice is to use a fully customized prosthesis made of any of the available artificial polymers, mimicking the contralateral side. Over the last few years, polyether ether ketone (PEEK) has been our material of choice, due to its great biocompatibility.

a

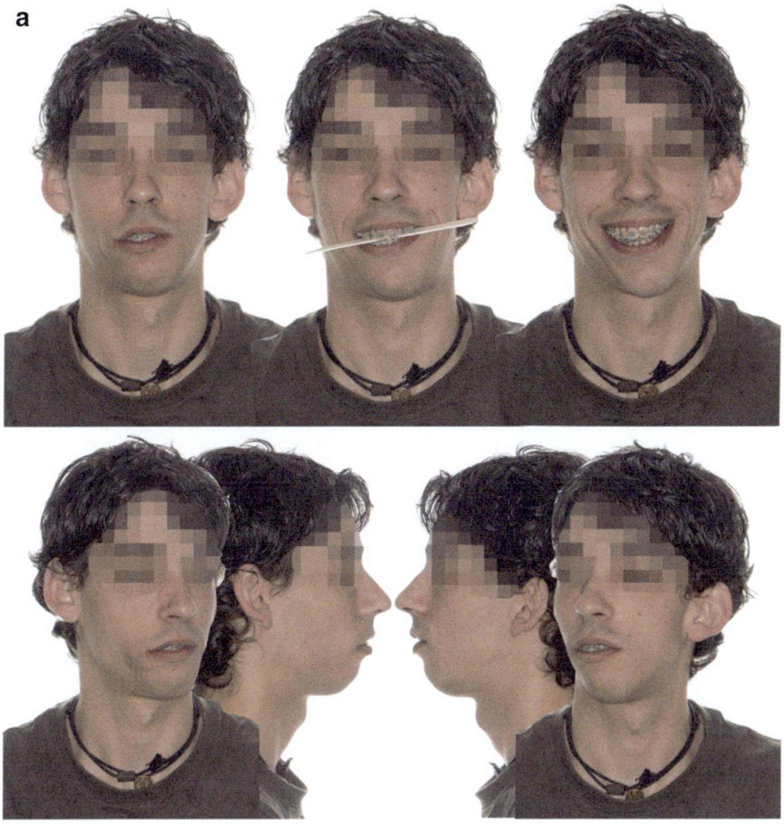

Fig. 5.2 (**a**) A 25-year-old patient who suffered an accident during childhood resulting in unnoticed condylar comminuted fracture. It subsequently provoked a severe facial deformity because of normal growth on the unaffected side of the mandible and vertical compensation from the maxilla, resulting in a severe maxillomandibular cant. (**b**) Three-dimensional planning for maxillomandibular surgery with asymmetry correction, counterclockwise rotation, and the design of a customized prosthesis to reconstruct the left temporomandibular joint and deficient ascending ramus. (**c**) Intraoperative views of the submandibular and preauricular access to install the prosthesis. (**d**) Presurgical and immediate postsurgical views. (**e**) Final result

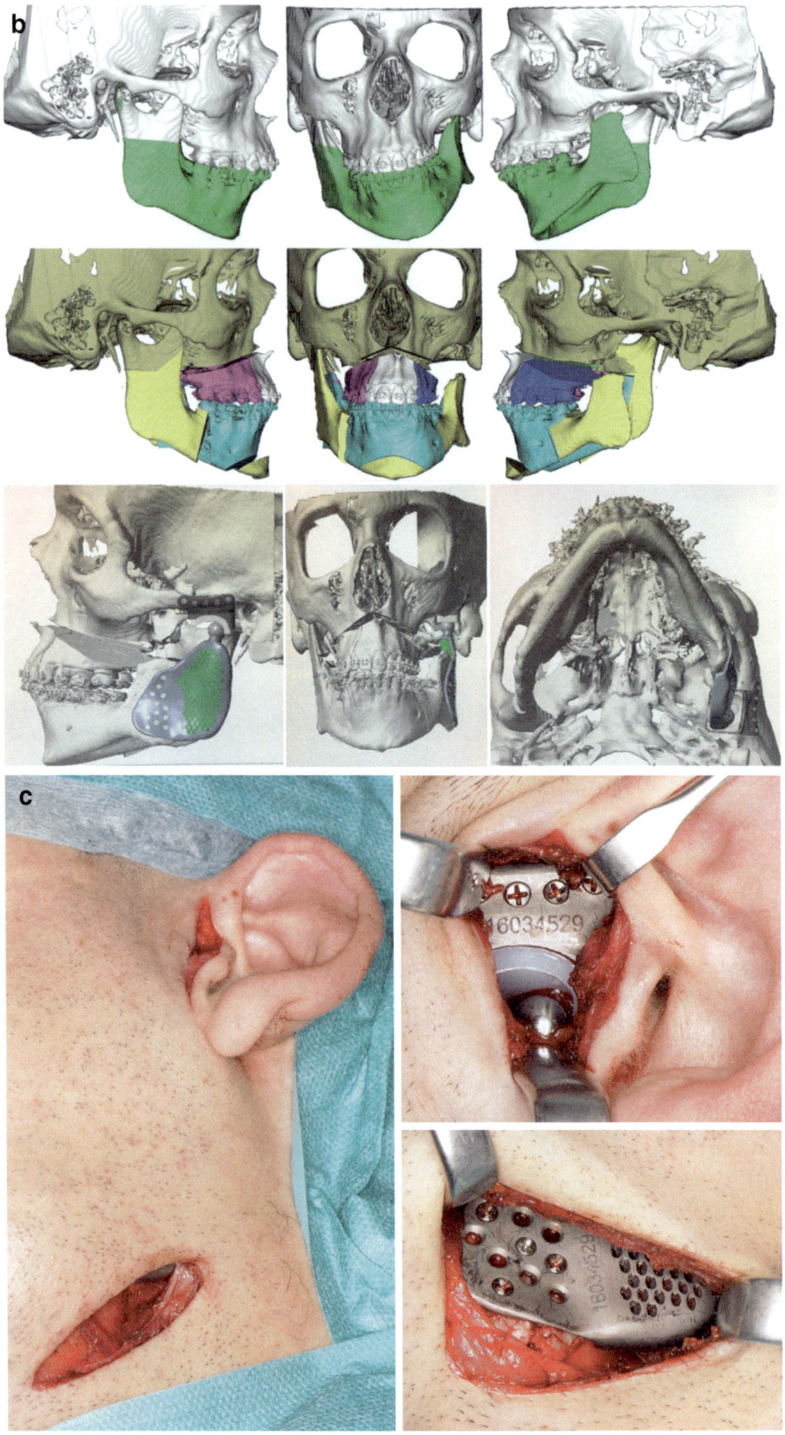

Fig. 5.2 (continued)

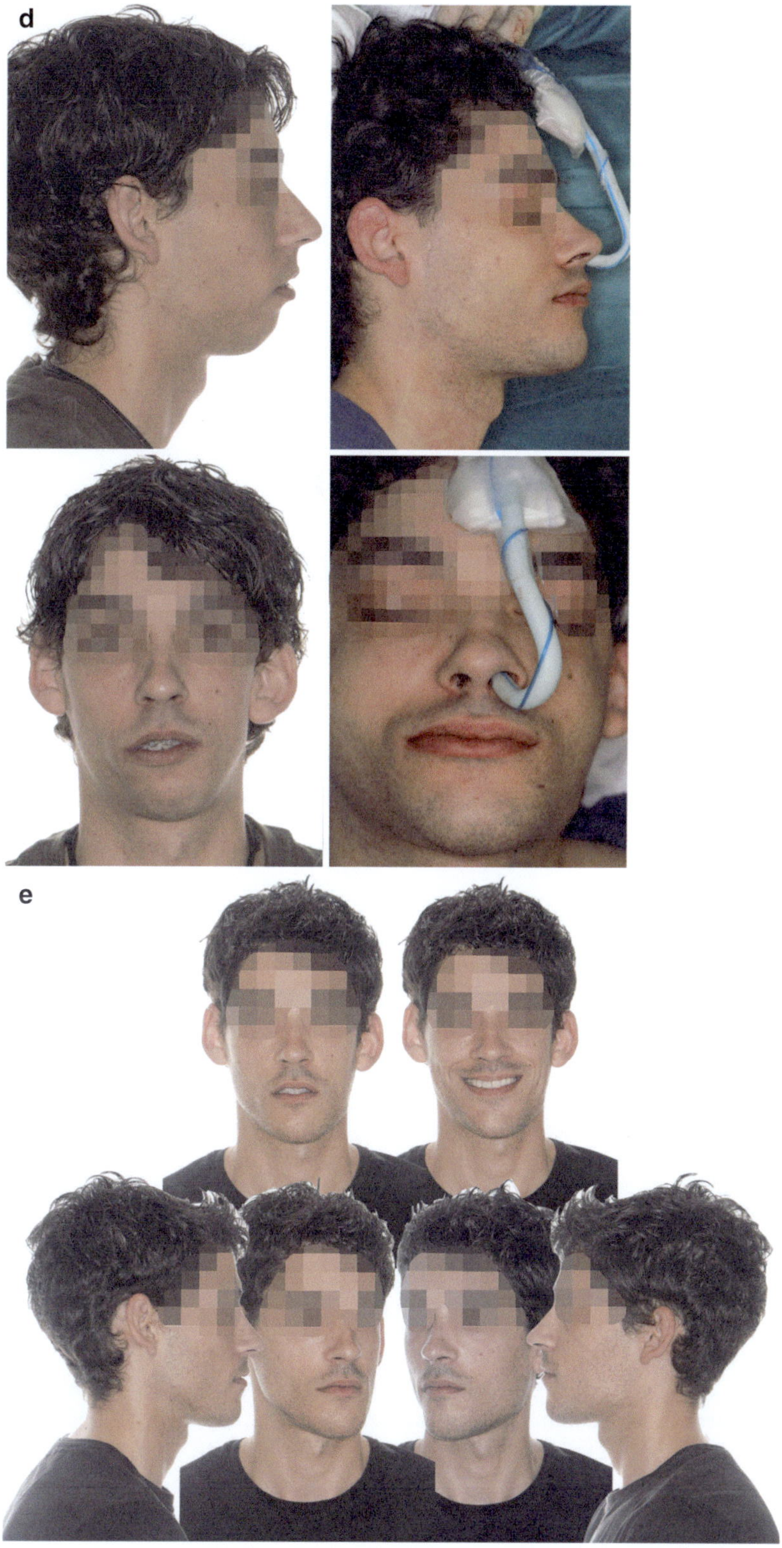

Fig. 5.2 (continued)

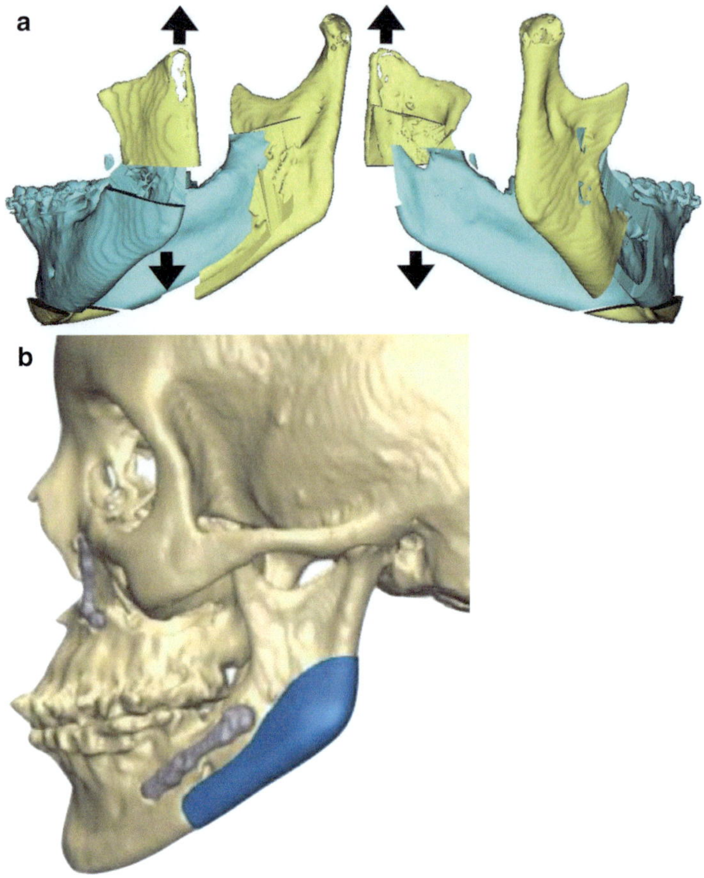

Fig. 5.3 (**a**) Modified Obwegeser osteotomy to allow elongation of the mandibular ramus. (**b**) Customized PEEK implant to achieve vertical symmetry of the mandibular ramus

5.2 Asymmetry Secondary to Unilateral Mandibular Overgrowth

Obwegeser [10, 11] proposed a classification of mandibular asymmetry secondary to excessive growth comprising two major groups according to the main vector on the excessive side.

5.2.1 Hemimandibular Elongation

In this situation, there is a predominant horizontal component, and the typical traits are

- Lower midline deviation.
- Cross-bite on the unaffected side.
- No or little canting of the occlusal plane.
- Class III occlusion on the affected side.
- Radiologically, the typical finding is elongation of the condyle and condylar neck (Fig. 5.4a and b).

5.2.2 Hemimandibular Hyperplasia

- No lower midline deviation.
- If secondary to fast condylar growth, open bite on the affected side.
- Canting of the occlusal plane.
- Typically, class I occlusion.
- Radiologically, the typical finding is a large and often amorphous (osteochondroma) condyle (Fig. 5.5a–d).

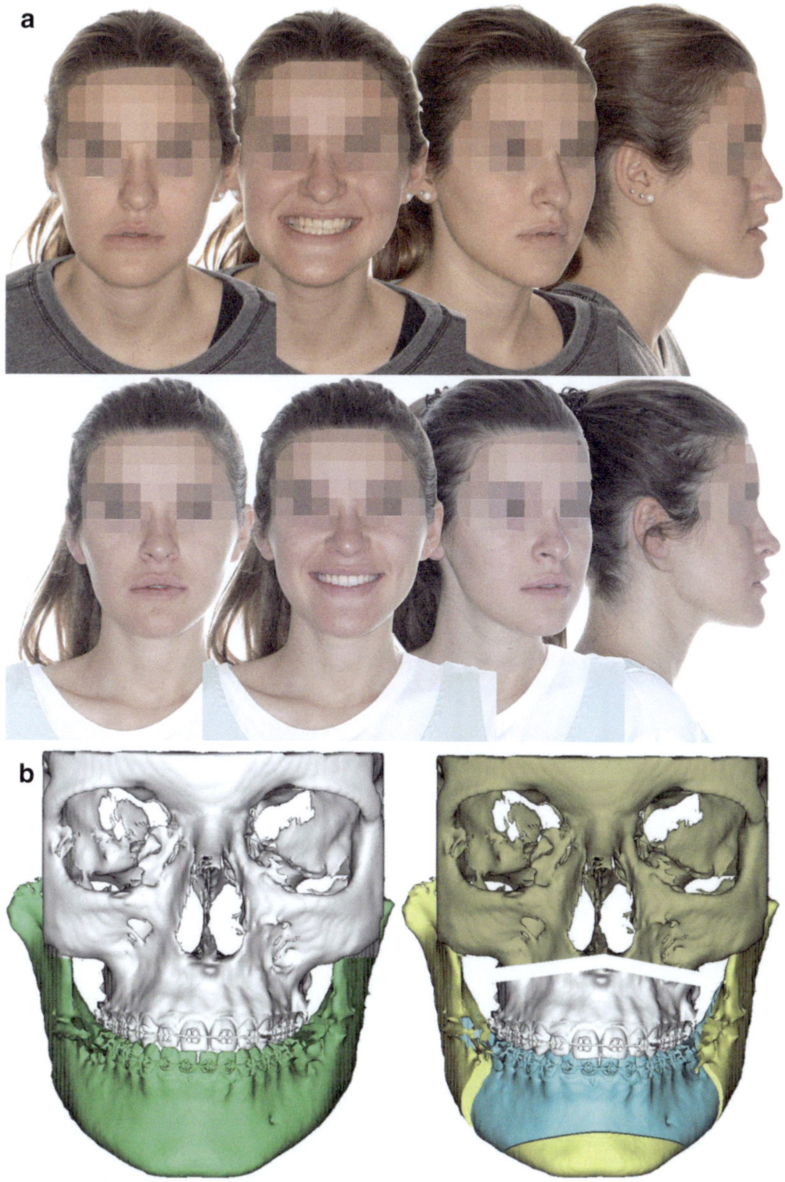

Fig. 5.4 (**a** and **b**) Facial asymmetry secondary to horizontal mandibular elongation managed with maxillomandibular surgery without intervention upon the temporomandibular joint

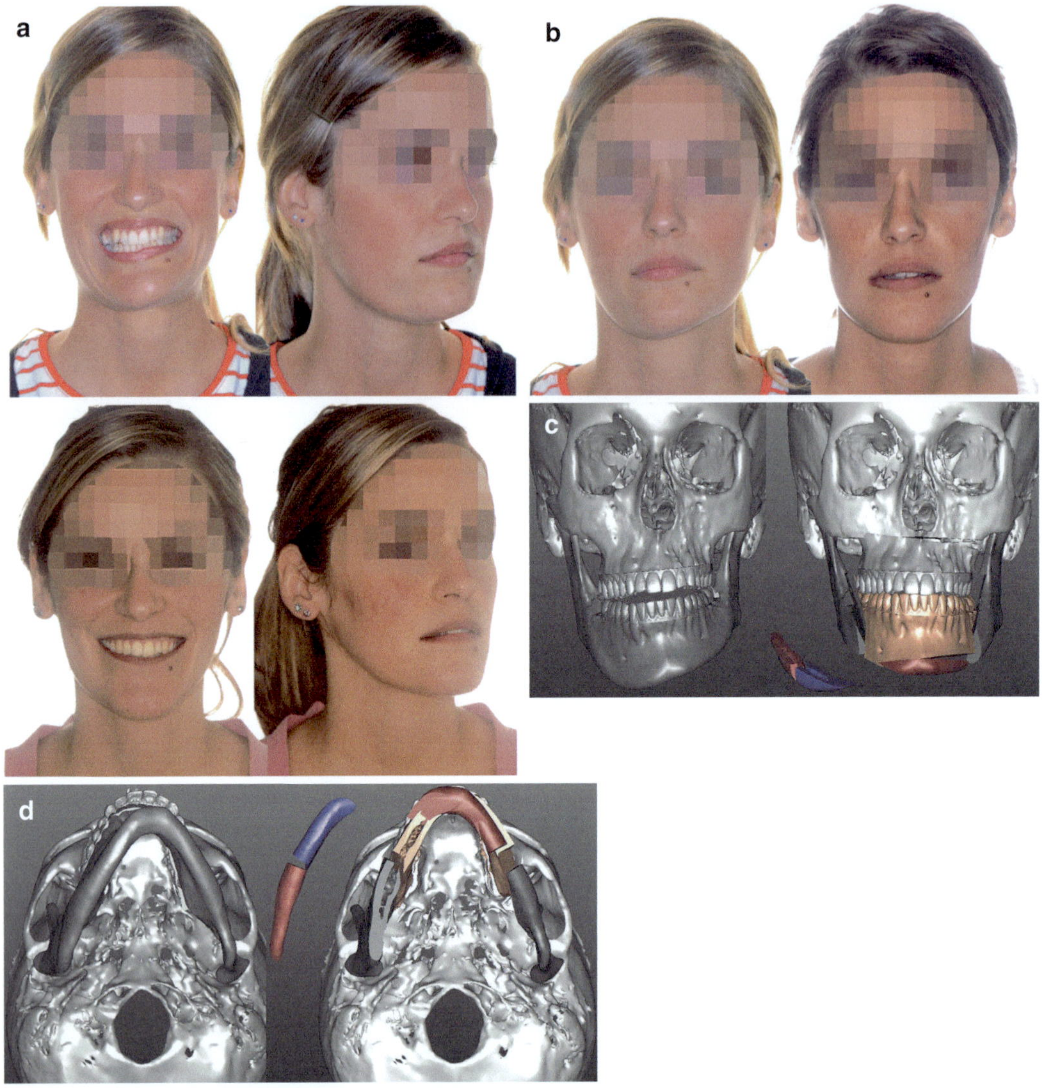

Fig. 5.5 (**a–d**) Facial asymmetry secondary to right condylar hyperplasia causing hemimandibular hypertrophy. This was managed via a simultaneous proportional condylectomy, BSSO, Le Fort I, and mandibular remodeling

In our experience, most cases are actually a mix of the previous forms because the clinical features are a sequel of the pathological growth of the condyle, being dependent mainly on the growth vector. Thus, if there is a more centered growth of the condyle, the sequelae will be more vertical with less horizontal components, while if there is a more medial or lateral growth of the condyle, the sequelae will be more horizontal with less vertical components, regardless of the type of disorder involved—condylar hyperplasia or condylar tumor (Fig. 5.6).

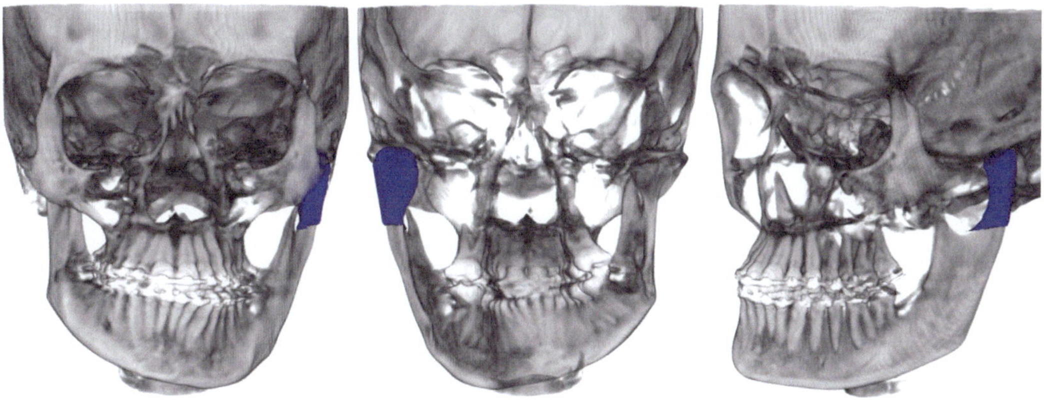

Fig. 5.6 Typical vertical growth compatible with either condylar hyperplasia or osteochondroma

5.3 Exact Timing of Surgery

Our protocol in asymmetrical patients consists of the following:

Growing or Young Patients We prefer to wait and see in these cases because in most circumstances the asymmetrical mandibular growth will cease spontaneously, and correction with orthognathic surgery will secure full correction once skeletal maturity is reached. The exception is pathological condylar situations because in these cases the preference is to perform condylectomy as soon as possible in order to avoid a severe asymmetrical condition, with vertical and horizontal components, causing open bite on the affected side and cross-bite on the contralateral side, plus maxillary canting.

Adults In the case of suspected active condylar growth with progressive facial deterioration or fast occlusal changes, scintigraphy will rule out condylar hyperplasia or a condylar tumor. If the combination of clinical changes and positive scintigraphy findings suggests high activity, a proportional condylectomy [12] should be performed, associated with orthognathic surgery in the event of facial asymmetry as a sequel (Fig. 5.7a–f).

CONDYLAR HYPERPLASIA APPROACH

ACTIVE GROWING CONDYLE			STOPPED GROWTH CONDYLE FACIAL ASSYMMETRY
FACIAL SIMMETRY	FACIAL ASSIMMETRY		
	GROWING PERIOD	ADULTHOOD	
WAIT & SEE	CONDYLAR SHAVING VS HIGH CONDYLECTOMY VS PROPORTIONAL CONDYLECTOMY	HIGH/ PROPORTIONAL CONDYLECTOMY +/- SURGICAL MANDIBULAR REPOSITIONING +/- ORTHODONTICS	ORTHODONTICS & SURGICAL MANDIBULAR REPOSITIONING +/-LE FORT I, INFERIOR BORDER OSTEOTOMY, GENIOPLASTY +/-CONDYLECTOMY

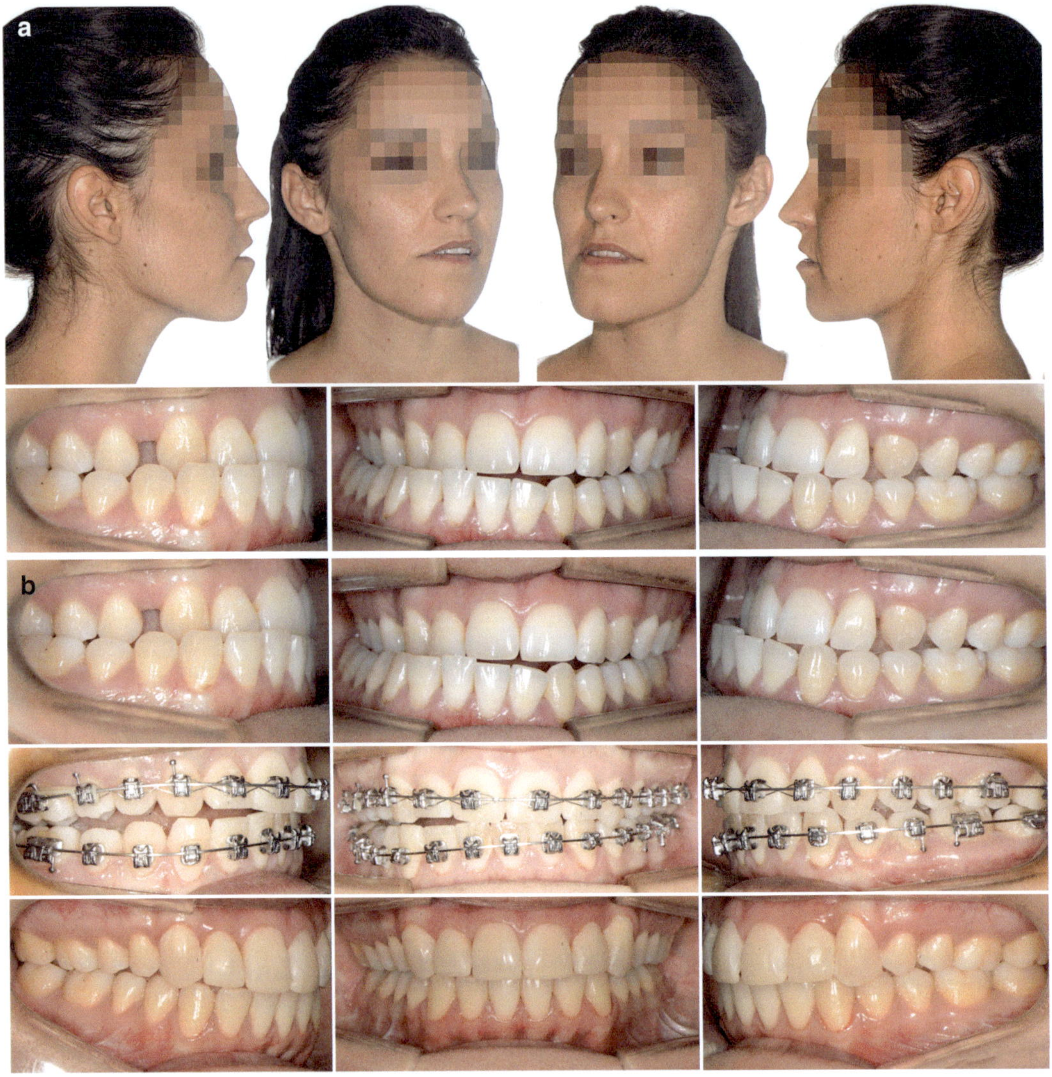

Fig. 5.7 (**a**–**f**) Severe vertical asymmetry secondary to left condylar osteochondroma. This was managed via condylectomy through an intraoral approach and bimaxillary surgery

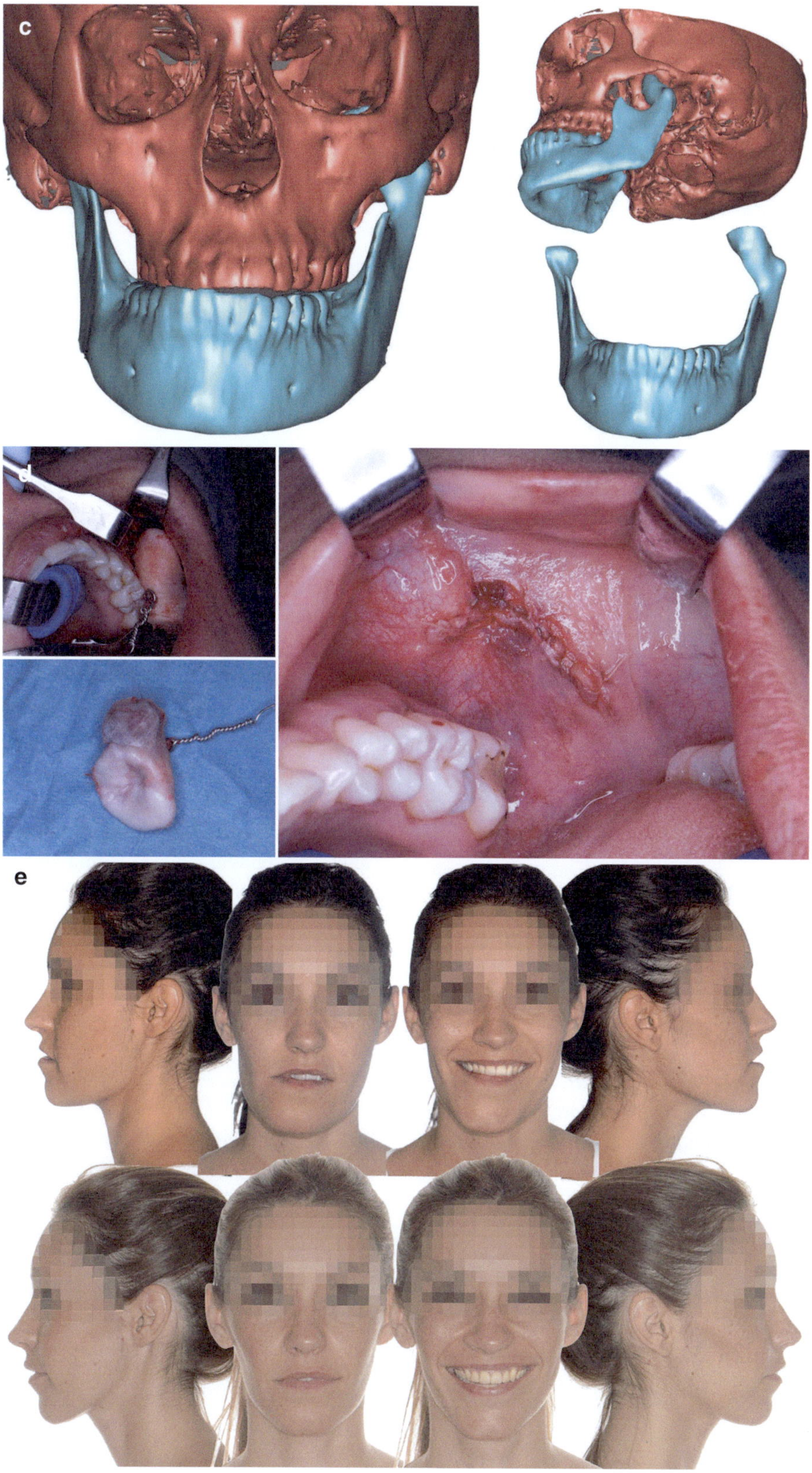

Fig. 5.7 (continued)

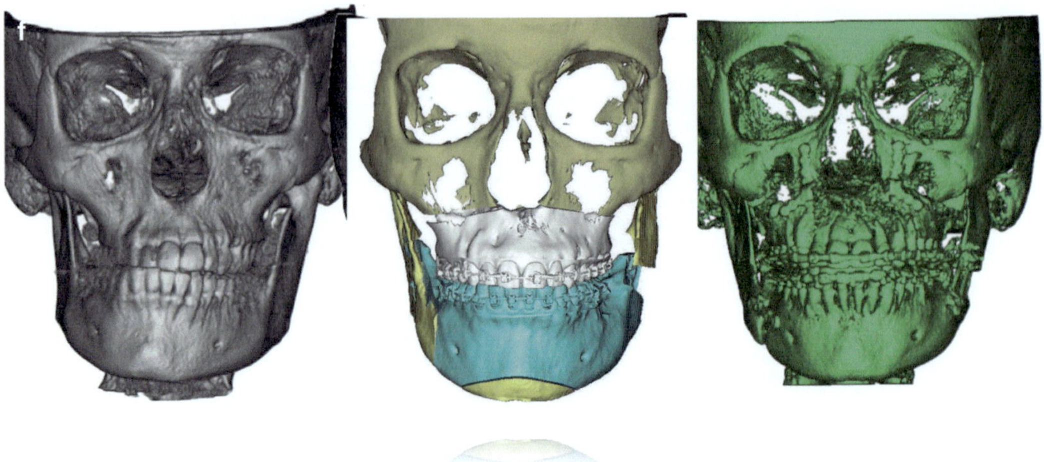

Fig. 5.7 (continued)

Treatment algorithm for patients with history of condylar hyperplasia, which mostly depends on the age of the patient, and presence of condylar activity and facial asymmetry

5.4 Condylectomy

Over the years, we have developed a condylectomy protocol involving a combination of techniques with a scientific basis. The main aspects are proportional condylectomy [12, 13], an intraoral approach to the pathological condyle [14], and a 3D-printed cutting guide [15].

We divide our protocol into two phases: virtual surgical planning and surgical approach.

Virtual Surgical Planning At this point, we create the virtual skull model as in orthognathic surgery for a better understanding of the condylar disorder and its repercussion upon the face. Planning begins with the virtual proportional condylectomy, where we measure both rami vertically; the excess of vertical ramus on the pathological side versus the healthy side is removed during surgery. The surgical simulation is done in the virtual environment. The ramus with the proportional condylectomy is exported from the Dolphin imaging software to the 3D Builder application (Windows 10, Microsoft Corporation, Redmond, WA, USA), where we design the 3D cutting guide in the sigmoid notch to the osteotomy region. The guide is manufactured with a 3D printer.

Surgical Approach The intraoral approach to the mandibular condyle is made with a small incision (2 cm) in the buccal mucosa in relation to the coronoid process. The mandibular ramus is exposed, and we detach the temporal muscle, gaining a subperiosteal access through the sigmoid notch to the condyle, entering the articular capsule and saving the soft tissue to a superior position. Thus, we have an intraoral view of the mandibular condyle. A maxillomandibular fixation (MMF) screw with a long steel wire is placed above the osteotomy region to facilitate removal of the hyperplastic segment. This is followed by insertion of the 3D-printed cutting guide in the best-fit position; osteotomy is performed with a piezoelectric tool, and the steel wire with the pathological condyle is removed. The sutures are resorbable. The entire surgical process tends to take about 25 min (Fig. 5.8a–c).

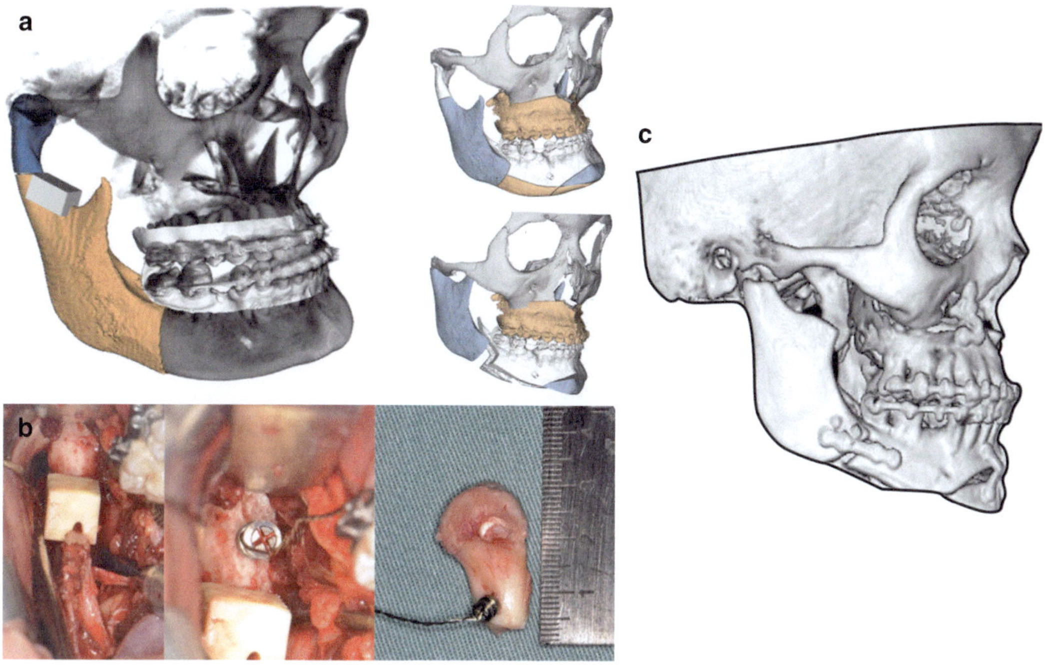

Fig. 5.8 (a–c) Intraoral proportional condylectomy aided by a customized cutting guide

5.5 Surgery Sequence in Hyperplastic Asymmetrical Patients

First, virtual planning is mandatory in asymmetrical patients. There is no good outcome without this tool. The procedure is important not only for planning but also for diagnosis [16–18].

Second, asymmetrical conditions are treated objectively in a frontal view. The midline, roll, and yaw must be measured, and both sides must be equal or at least proportionally symmetrical in the 3D virtual planning software (Fig. 5.9).

In relation to surgical timing, we usually perform mandible first. Exceptions are when there is a pathological condition requiring condylectomy or a maxillary cant requiring a large maxillary upward surgical movement on one of the sides. Thus, our surgical sequence is as follows:

Regular Facial Asymmetry We always perform mandible first, centering the jaw and using it as a reference for the position of the maxilla and chin.

Sequence—Mandible/Maxilla/Chin

Facial Asymmetry with Condylar Pathology Proportional condylectomy should be performed as a first step, with the mandible after that. It is important to have a fixed region as a reference after condylectomy because the mandible will change position. We therefore do not perform maxilla first under these conditions.

Sequence—Proportional condylectomy/Mandible/Maxilla/Chin

Facial Asymmetry with Great Maxillary Canting Maxilla is performed first to avoid inadequate fixation of the mandible and consequently inaccurate surgery. When a large upward surgical movement of the maxilla is necessary, if we perform mandible first, it is difficult to know the correct position for fixing the jaw, since it will be fixed with the rotation of the proximal segment; as a result, the mandible cannot occupy an upward position if the maxilla has not yet been operated upon (Fig. 5.10a–h).

Sequence—Maxilla/Mandible/Chin

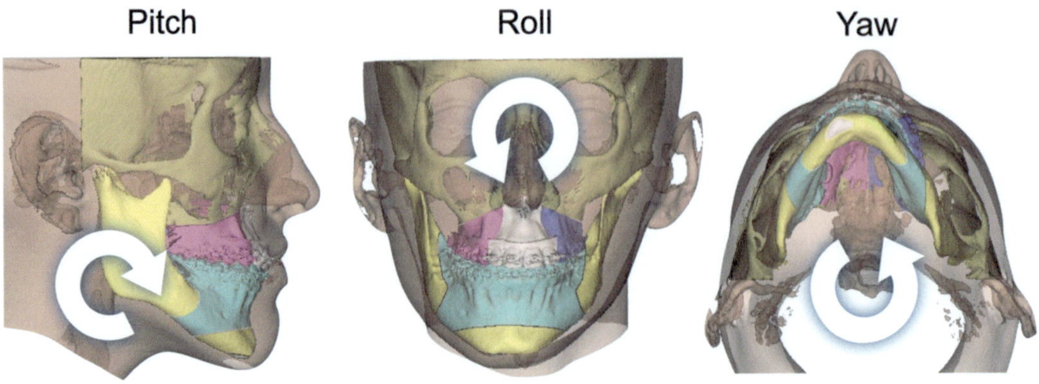

Fig. 5.9 Virtual planning in asymmetries must incorporate pitch, yaw, and roll corrections

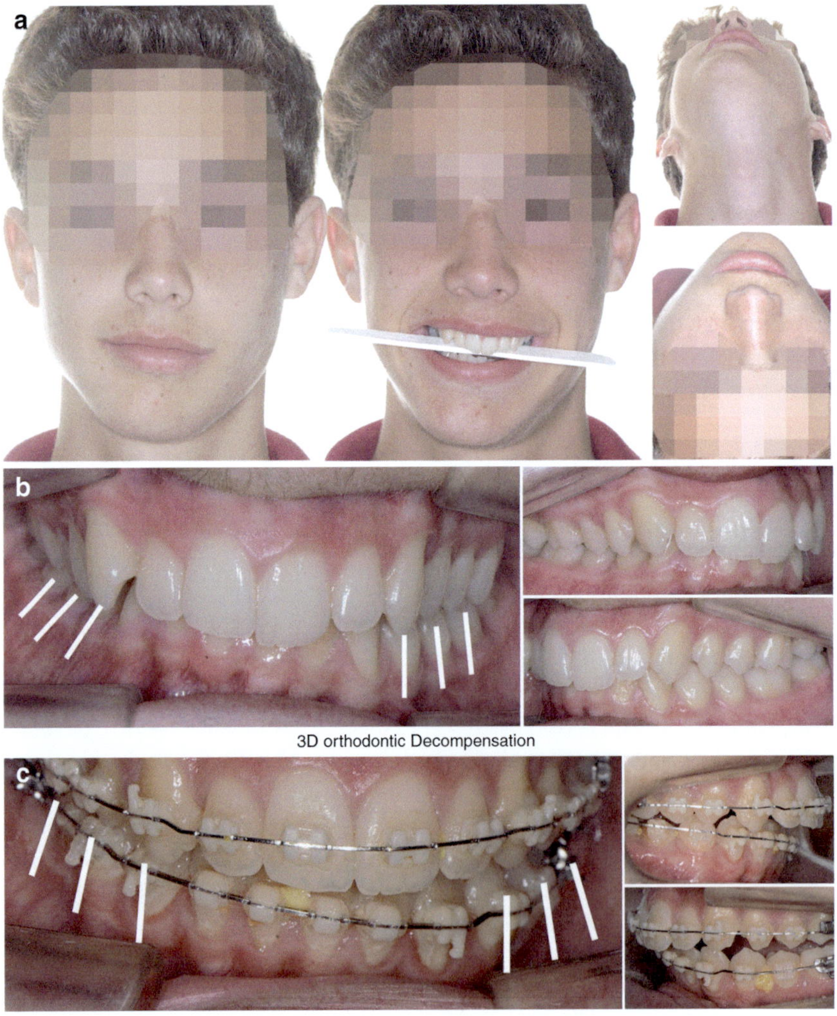

Fig. 5.10 (a–h) Severe facial asymmetry due to early-onset right condylar hypoplasia managed with 3D orthodontic decompensation and bimaxillary surgery in which a "maxilla first" protocol was used

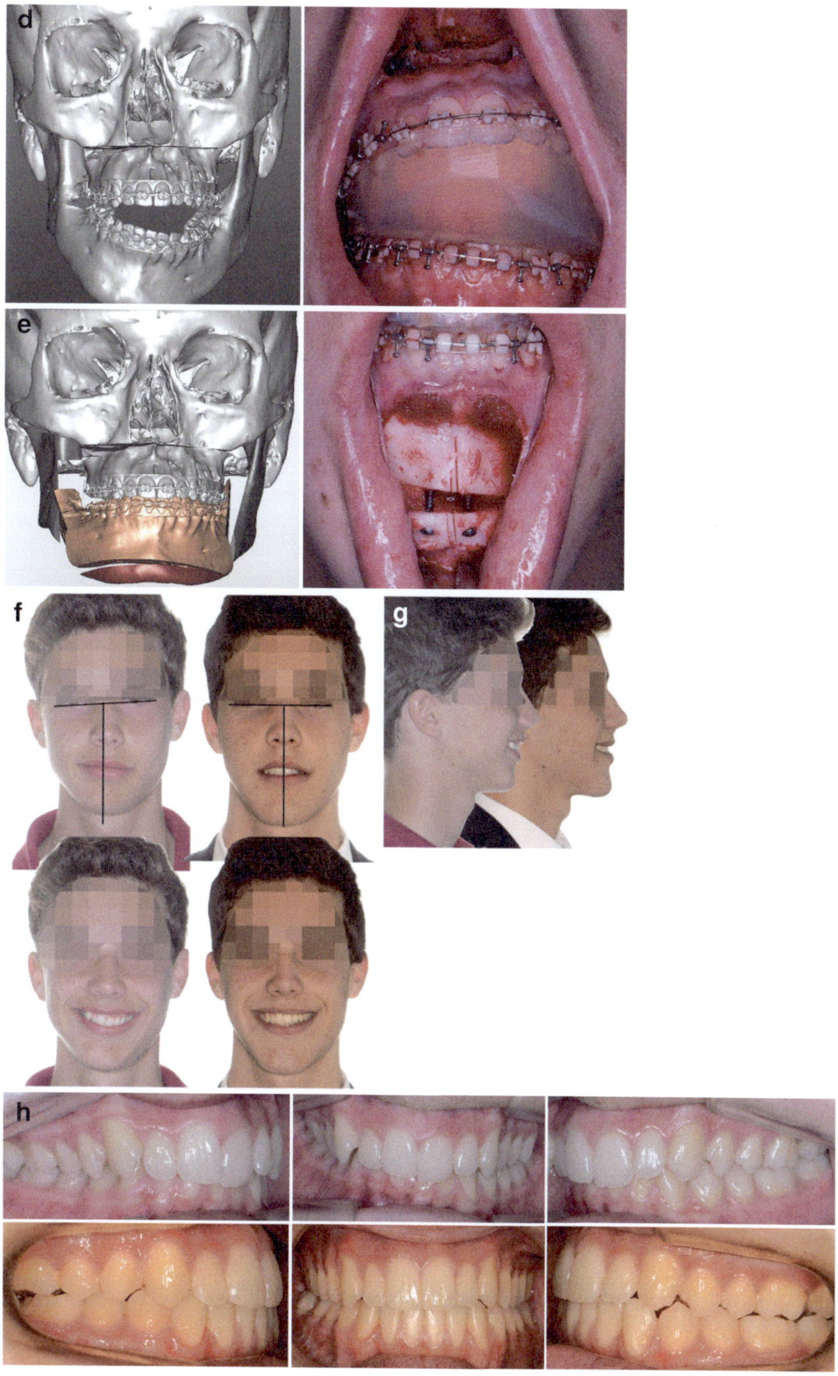

Fig. 5.10 (continued)

References

1. Xue Z, Wu L, Qiu T, Li Z, Wang X, Liu X. Three-dimensional dynamic analysis of the facial movement symmetry of skeletal class III patients with facial asymmetry. J Oral Maxillofac Surg. 2020;78(2):267–74.
2. Duran GS, Taşdelen FÖ, Dindaroğlu F. Effect of facial profile convexity on the perception of mandibular asymmetry using three-dimensional stereophotogrammetric images. Orthod Craniofac Res. 2020;23(1):110–7.
3. Chen YJ, Yao CC, Chang ZC, Lai HH, Yeh KJ, Kok SH. Characterization of facial asymmetry in skeletal Class III malocclusion and its implications for treatment. Int J Oral Maxillofac Surg. 2019;48(12):1533–41.
4. López DF, Botero JR, Muñoz JM, Cárdenas-Perilla R, Moreno M. Are there mandibular morphological differences in the various facial asymmetry etiologies? A tomographic three-dimensional reconstruction study. J Oral Maxillofac Surg. 2019;77(11):2324–38.
5. Evangelista K, de Oliveira CFP, de Almeida BL, Avelino MAG, Cevidanes LHS, de Oliveira Ruellas AC, Valladares-Neto J, Silva MAG. Three-dimensional assessment of craniofacial asymmetry in children with transverse maxillary deficiency after rapid maxillary expansion: a prospective study. Orthod Craniofac Res. 2020. [Epub ahead of print];23:300.
6. Thiesen G, Gribel BF, Freitas MPM, Oliver DR, Kim KB. Mandibular asymmetries and associated factors in orthodontic and orthognathic surgery patients. Angle Orthod. 2018;88(5):545–51.
7. Bernini JM, Kellenberger CJ, EichenbergerM ET, Papageorgiou SN, Patcas R. Quantitative analysis of facial asymmetry based on three-dimensional photography: a valuable indicator for asymmetrical temporomandibular joint affection in juvenile idiopathic arthritis patients? Pediatric Rheumatology. 2020;18(1):Article Number 10.
8. Stoustrup P, Pedersen TK, Nørholt SE, Resnick CM, Abramowicz S. Interdisciplinary management of dentofacial deformity in juvenile idiopathic arthritis. Oral Maxillofac Surg Clin North Am. 2020;32(1):117–34.
9. Peacock ZS, Lee CCY, Troulis MJ, Kaban LB. Long-term stability of condylectomy and costochondral graft reconstruction for treatment of idiopathic condylar resorption. J Oral Maxillofac Surg. 2019;77(4):792–802.
10. Obwegeser HL, Makek MS. Hemimandibular hyperplasia—hemimandibular elongation. J Maxillofac Surg. 1986;14(4):183–208.
11. Obwegeser HL, Obwegeser JA. New clinical-based evidence for the existence of 2 growth regulators in mandibular condyles: hemimandibular elongation in hemifacial microsomia mandible. J Craniofac Surg. 2010;21(5):1595–600.
12. Fariña R, Moreno E, Lolas J, Silva F, Martínez B. Three-dimensional skeletal changes after early proportional condylectomy for condylar hyperplasia. Int J Oral Maxillofac Surg. 2019;48:941–51.
13. Fariña R, Olate S, Raposo A, Araya I, Alister JP, Uribe F. High condylectomy versus proportional condylectomy: is secondary orthognathic surgery necessary? Int J Oral Maxillofac Surg. 2016;45:72–7.
14. Hernández-Alfaro F, Méndez-Manjón I, Valls-Ontañón A, Guijarro-Martínez R. Minimally invasive intraoral condylectomy: proof of concept report. Int J Oral Maxillofac Surg. 2016;45(9):1108–14.
15. Haas Junior OL, Fariña R, Hernández-Alfaro F, de Oliveira RB. Minimally invasive intraoral proportional condylectomy with 3D-printed cutting guide. Int J Oral Maxillofac Surg. 2020. [Epub ahead of print];49:1435.
16. Hernández-Alfaro F, Guijarro-Martínez R. New protocol for three-dimensional surgical planning and CAD/CAM splint generation in orthognathic surgery: an in vitro and in vivo study. Int J Oral Maxillofac Surg. 2013;42(12):1547–56.
17. Aboul-Hosn Centenero S, Hernández-Alfaro F. 3D planning in orthognathic surgery: CAD/CAM surgical splints and prediction of the soft and hard tissues results e our experience in 16 cases. J Craniofac Surg. 2012;40(2):162–8.
18. Haas OL Jr, Becker OE, de Oliveira RB. Computer-aided planning in orthognathic surgery—systematic review. Int J Oral Maxillofac Surg. 2015;44:329–42.

Surgical Orthodontics

6

Juan Carlos Pérez Varela, Miriam López Vila, and Laura González García

6.1 Introduction

In order to provide our patients with the highest quality of care, we diagnose and design treatment plans that will enable us to determine whether they should undergo orthodontic treatment alone or orthodontic treatment combined with surgery. The surgical and orthodontic approaches have been shown to be very effective in treating deformities of the dentofacial region that cannot be concealed by orthodontic treatment alone. Combining model analysis, space analysis, cephalometric analysis, photoanalysis, and soft-tissue analysis can provide us with a detailed treatment plan that meets the orthodontic goals for facial and dental aesthetics, function, occlusion, and periodontal health. The orthodontist plays an important role in this multidisciplinary approach throughout the various phases of treatment, including treatment evaluation, presurgical orthodontics, orthognathic surgery, and postsurgical orthodontics.

J. C. Pérez Varela · M. L. Vila (✉) · L. G. García
Orthodontic Clinic Dr Juan Carlos Pérez Varela, Calle Doctor Teixeiro, Santiago de Compostela (A coruña), Spain

6.2 Presurgical Orthodontics

6.2.1 Presurgical Goals

Most nonorthodontic patients who have skeletal discrepancies between the mandible and maxilla do not have their dental arches leveled. As a consequence, irregularities on the occlusal plane may interfere with the placement of teeth at certain points during surgical jaw relocation, reducing the possibility of placing them in their optimal position [1, 2]. Presurgical occlusion therefore dictates surgical movements, which, in the worst case scenario, are restricted as a consequence [3]. Presurgical orthodontics aims to achieve optimal skeletal correction by aligning and leveling the arch prior to surgery. The essential steps in orthodontic preparation for orthognathic surgery include

1. Teeth alignment and leveling without concern for occlusion.
2. Anterior–posterior and vertical positioning of the incisors.
3. Achievement of arch compatibility [4].

Improper planning may result in poor surgical results and a longer postoperative period. The time required for preoperative orthodontics is typically 15–17 months, and sometimes even longer. Approximately 7–12 months are required for the postoperative orthodontic phase [5, 6].

F. Hernández-Alfaro, A. Valls Ontañón (eds.), *Orthofacial Surgery*,
https://doi.org/10.1007/978-3-031-76185-0_6

For such poor outcomes to be avoided, a thorough understanding of tooth movement is required prior to the procedure. It is therefore necessary to plan the following:

1. The position of the teeth anteroposteriorly, vertically, and transversally
2. How to position these teeth or tooth segments, surgically or orthodontically, to maximize the speed and efficacy of treatment [6]

6.2.2 Arch Alignment

In preparation for surgery, the level, alignment, spacing, and crowding of both arches should be assessed. When correcting dental crowding, we must take into account that the inclination of the incisors will increase, and for surgical preparation, it is essential to normalize this [7].

When the above occurs, there are several treatment alternatives. If the inclination is slight, stripping may be sufficient, but when it is moderate or severe, it is usually necessary to resort to premolar extractions or the use of microscrews for distalization in combination with the extraction of the wisdom teeth (which is often necessary also for orthognathic surgery itself).

If extractions are needed, they should be performed 6 months before surgery. This allows the bone to heal and fill, preventing a bad split and facilitating surgery [8]. During this phase, the closing of spaces is not our priority. Therefore, sometimes, an amount of spacing may be desirable at the time of surgery in order to provide greater overjet for proper placement of the canine at the time of surgery or to accommodate postoperative leveling without forward movement of the lower incisors [7].

6.2.2.1 Leveling of the Arches

Leveling is done by intrusion–extrusion. Leveling or not leveling the lower arch before surgery has a significant impact upon the final position of the chin and the height of the lower face after surgery [4, 7] and is necessary to achieve a stable postoperative occlusion.

6.2.3 Dental Decompensations

Dental compensations are defined as alterations in the normal axial inclinations and vertical position that may occur in response to disharmonious skeletal growth. They occur in the three planes of space: anteroposterior, vertical, and transversal [9].

The treatment plan should take into account possible post-treatment changes that may have an adverse impact upon stability. Ideally, orthodontic movements should be designed in such a manner that any orthodontic change will occur in the opposite direction to the anticipated surgical change. For example, in the case of an open bite, the preferred movement is to intrude the incisors forward prior to surgery to balance any skeletal tendency toward open bite recurrence after treatment [7].

During presurgical orthodontic preparation, it is essential to carry out radiographic controls to assess the improvement of dental inclinations and plaster models or to print in three dimensions to control postsurgical occlusion.

To improve occlusion before surgery, it is often necessary to use intermaxillary elastics, which can also help improve dental inclinations.

In class III occlusion cases, class II elastics are used to decompensate the retroinclined mandibular incisors and proclined maxillary incisors, while class III elastics are recommended for class II cases [8].

Nevertheless, we must remember that controlling the anchorage is crucial, since presurgical orthodontic treatment is based on a stable mandibular position. Therefore, we often must resort to intra-arch mechanisms instead of intermaxillary mechanisms; in this case, temporary anchorage devices (TADs) such as mini-screws or mini-plates can be of great help [1].

Temporary anchorage devices have opened up an array of new anchoring possibilities in orthodontics, with increased orthodontic efficiency and reduced treatment times. Temporary anchorage devices can be used in presurgical preparation and also in postsurgical control for different functions; for example, in maxillary segmentation, TADs are used for vertical control anteriorly and for vertical and transverse control posteriorly [5]. They also may be beneficial in cases of skeletal class II malocclusion, where the maxillary dentition must be moved backward or the mandibular molars must be moved forward, in order to achieve the desired occlusion. In skeletal class III cases, TADs distalize the entire mandibular dentition [10] and are also widely used today in the postsurgical control of patients treated with aligners, etc.

As a result of temporary occlusion and facial profile degradation during presurgical treatment, patients who undergo dental decompensation are believed to have lower oral health-related quality of life. It is therefore important to warn patients that in this early phase, their skeletal problems will be exaggerated aesthetically, functionally, and occlusally [11].

6.2.4 Arch Coordination

It is essential to achieve adequate coordination of the dental arches, for although the dental fit must continue to improve after surgery, it is necessary to have occlusion that is as stable as possible for postsurgical orthodontic control.

As we have explained above, in order to coordinate the arches, it is necessary to align and level the teeth and, of course, correct the dental inclinations.

Likewise, during the preparation, it is necessary to carry out model controls to assess the improvement of the occlusion, i.e., of the coordination of the arches during the preparation.

To perform such an assessment, we must place the models in a class I dental relationship and in that position assess the dental interferences and how to correct them. For this, we make use of orthodontic archwires, microscrews, intermaxillary elastics, etc., and assess the improvement by repeating these models with the frequency considered necessary according to the movements to be carried out.

Of course, we must take into account those cases in which there is maxillary compression. When the transverse problem is very slight, it can be compensated with intermaxillary elastics, thus avoiding a segmented Le Fort procedure, when the maxillary compression is less than 7 mm (the best way to assess this is by measuring it on a cone-beam computed tomography [CBCT] scan). Likewise, of course, and as long as the maxillofacial surgeon agrees, we could perform orthognathic surgery with a segmented Le Fort procedure and, when the maxillary compression is greater than 7 mm, surgically assisted rapid palatal expansion (SARPE) is required prior to orthognathic surgery.

The best way to assess the severity of maxillary compression is first to transversely decompensate the lower arch (since in cases with maxillary compression, there is usually negative transverse torque of the lower teeth) and then measure it on a CBCT scan.

There are different ways to perform such measurement. For example, it can be made from the center of the alveolus of the right molar to the center of the alveolus of the left molar, in both the upper and the lower arches, or from the outermost part of the bone at the level of the first molars, both upper and lower [12]. The objective we must keep in mind is that the upper arch should measure crosswise about 4–5 mm more than the lower one and, according to this criterion, we will determine the need for maxillary expansion to later assess the most appropriate way to achieve it.

In the case of the segmented Le Fort procedure, the most common strategy is to perform segmentation between the lateral incisor and the canine. It is therefore essential to place the roots parallel to each other and even, whenever possible, open a space of at least 2 mm on each side between these teeth to reduce the risk of damaging one when segmenting.

On the other hand, when it is necessary to carry out prior SARPE, we perform a first orthodontic phase to decompensate the lower arch. This phase usually lasts between 4 and 6 months; later, SARPE will be carried out with a bone-supported expander (we use the Power Expander by Pérez-Varela®), and 1 month later, after completing expansion, the upper teeth will begin to move to close the diastema and continue the preparation for orthognathic surgery (in the clinical case of this chapter, we will explain this procedure in more detail).

6.3 Treatment Planning

Once all the presurgical objectives have been reached (alignment, leveling, dental decompensation, and coordination of the arches), the patient is ready to undergo surgery.

In order for the intervention to be as exact as possible, virtual planning must be carried out in advance, establishing a tentative postsurgical result and, in that ideal final position, acrylic guides are made so that when performing surgery, they help the maxillofacial surgeon to perform the skeletal movements as close as possible to the virtually determined position. Surgical guides are helpful during sagittal and transverse movements but not for vertical movements.

To perform planning, it is necessary to take a series of records once the patient has been prepared, and from that moment until after surgery, no more dental movements should be made, for otherwise the guides could become misaligned.

The necessary records are: intraoral and extraoral photographs, teleradiography, CBCT scan, and intraoral scanning.

There are various software applications for carrying out virtual planning in which the CBCT scan, intraoral scanning, and the extraoral photographs are superimposed and, subsequently, the necessary skeletal movements are performed virtually.

To determine the amount and type of movement each patient needs, there are different aesthetic references. Our recommendation in planning sagittal movements is to use the aesthetic line that passes through the soft nasion perpendicular to the Frankfurt line and, in general, the goal will be for the nasal spine to be located at 1.07 ± 3.70 mm and point B at −6.87 ± 5.88 mm with respect to this line—though of course there are other anatomical points that we must take into account [13].

In addition, we must center the upper and lower dental lines with the aesthetic midline of the face, normalize facial height and overbite, asymmetries of the jaws and, in cases where there is a transverse problem, plan the millimeters of expansion necessary to solve it (in segmented Le Fort, the expansion should not be greater than 7 mm; in this case, the ideal approach is to perform prior SARPE).

The objective of the jaw movements will always be to improve the occlusion, function, health, and aesthetics of the patient.

It is important to add that with the advancement in orthognathic surgery, there is always improvement of the airway of the patients, which is especially important in individuals who suffer from previous problems of this type.

6.4 Surgery

As we have explained above, orthognathic surgery is performed by the maxillofacial surgeon with the help of virtual planning and previously made guides.

In preparation for orthognathic surgery with brackets, full-dimension stainless steel orthodontic arch wires are placed. It is intended that these arch wires will withstand the use of heavy elastics during the postoperative orthodontic treatment phase in order to refine any minor skeletal movements and counterbalance any soft tissue pull that may lead to relapse [2].

In cases with aligners, as previously explained, microscrews will be placed (their position will be determined according to the patient needs) before or during surgery, plus buttons on the teeth, to facilitate postsurgical control with intermaxillary elastics.

6.5 Postsurgical Orthodontics

Generally, the patient should return to the orthodontist approximately 1 week later to begin postsurgical treatment with intermaxillary elastics. The first day, soft elastics are used, and little by little, their strength and number are increased; the time will depend on the recovery of each individual patient and on the skeletal consolidation after surgery.

Our patients are advised to follow a soft diet for the first week and then gradually progress to foods that require more chewing. Six to eight weeks after surgery, a normal diet should be restored. During the first week after surgery, the patients should open and close their mouth as comfortably as possible. For the next 2 weeks, three 10–15 min sessions of opening and closing, combined with lateral movements, are recommended. Normal range of motion is expected 8 weeks after surgery [4].

During this final phase, our primary goals are to stabilize the skeletal movements and detail and finish the dental occlusion.

It is important to explain that in cases where the segmented Le Fort procedure is performed, an occlusal or palatal splint will be placed between the upper and lower arches, as well as intermaxillary elastics, to provide stability.

In cases where palatal expansion has been minimal, the splint may be removed 1–2 months after the procedure. For maxillary expansion greater than 3–4 mm, the splint should be worn for at least 2 or even 3 months, or longer if necessary. Following removal, post-orthodontic retainers, removable palatal splints, or heavy labial arches can be worn to maintain the maxillary expansions [14].

Of course, as in any medical intervention, there are risks and possible complications that may appear after the intervention, some immediately and others later on. When this happens, it is essential to identify them and address them as soon as possible.

A successful treatment begins with effective communication. An accurate skeletal diagnosis and treatment plan between the orthodontist and the surgeon will help to prevent unforeseen outcomes that may cause the treatment to be extended or increase frustration for all parties. Failure to accomplish this may result in complications such as insufficient or improvised dental decompensation, delay or increase of the magnitude of the operation more than intended, and a less than satisfactory skeletal and aesthetic result. Therefore, it is very important to emphasize tooth decompensation to make dental discrepancy as close to skeletal discrepancy as possible, eliminate dental interferences that may prevent optimal occlusion, and take into account tooth size discrepancies that may prevent the desired postoperative overjet or overbite. In those cases where optimal occlusion cannot be achieved after surgery, it is essential to determine whether the problem could be solved with orthodontics or if surgical reintervention would be necessary (a larger postoperative cephalogram and temporomandibular joint tomography would be useful). In addition, orthodontic appliances may also cause complications. During surgery, it is crucial that the appliances be securely attached to the teeth in order to minimize the risk of brackets being separated from the teeth. In order to avoid the possibility of dislodging of the wire and dissolving into the wound, bands are recommended for distal molars. Moreover, tooth movement should not occur within 8 weeks prior to surgery, as this may result in unintended intraoperative occlusion. Postoperative complications such as infections, exposure of titanium plates, or mobility may be a result of unrecognized or untreated temporomandibular joint pathology [14, 15].

In cases where repeat surgery is necessary, the surgeon will determine the most appropriate time according to skeletal healing, and in some cases, muscle deprogramming with an offloading splint and physiotherapy will be necessary to bring the joint into centric relation.

6.6 Clinical Case

A 25-year-old male with skeletal class II occlusion, maxillary compression, mandibular asymmetry, severe open bite, temporomandibular joint pain, bruxism, oral respiration, atypical swallowing habit, and severe dental crowding visited the orthodontic clinic to improve his smile and facial aesthetics.

The frontal clinical examination revealed a dolichofacial face, with mandibular deviation to the left, an important anterior open bite and buccal corridors due to a transverse problem of the maxilla, and a lack of positive transverse torque of the upper teeth. Profile evaluation revealed a concave profile (Figs. 6.1 and 6.2).

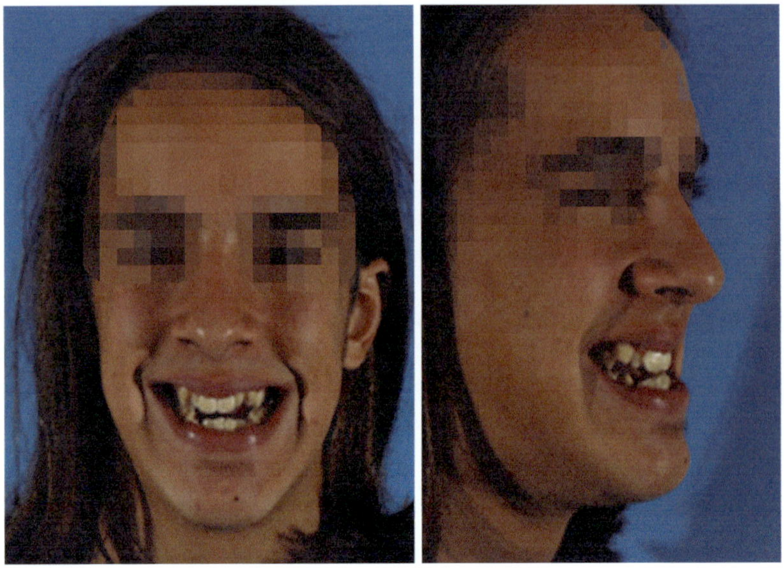

Fig. 6.1 Pretreatment extraoral views

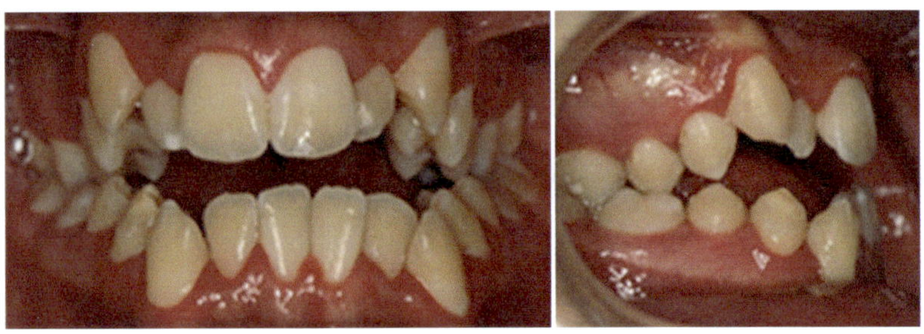

Fig. 6.2 Pretreatment intraoral views

Temporomandibular joint (TMJ) examination revealed pain in the joint.

In the teleradiographic study, we can observe class II occlusion and adequate inclination of the lower incisors (Fig. 6.3), though by aligning the lower arch, the inclination of the incisors will increase, and we will have to normalize it later on.

6.6.1 Treatment Progress

Once the clinical, photographic, and radiographic studies had been carried out, the patient was offered the following options:

A. Orthodontic compensation: Not recommended, due to the skeletal problems of the patient, which would not be corrected, and because of the long-term stability of the open bite.
B. SARPE and TADs: We would correct the maxillary transverse problem, reduce class III occlusion as much as possible, and close the open bite with the help of TADs and intermaxillary elastics, but we will not solve the asymmetry.
C. Orthognathic surgery (with previous SARPE): This was the ideal option, as we would correct all the skeletal and dental problems.

The patient decided to accept treatment option C. In this case, it was necessary to perform SARPE prior to orthognathic surgery because the required expansion exceeded 7 mm, and the surgeon agreed to perform it in two surgeries.

To begin, a first phase was carried out involving the placement of lower brackets to correctly position the teeth and an upper splint to relax the muscles and make sure the temporomandibular joint was in centric relation. This phase lasted 3–5 months.

In addition to correcting the alignment and leveling the lower arch, in preparation for SARPE, it is essential to adequately decompensate the arch transversally in order to subsequently perform maxillary expansion in the most precise way possible (Fig. 6.4).

When performing dental decompensation, in this first phase of treatment, the aesthetic problems in the patient's smile also became more evident, making the transverse maxillary problem, the open bite, and the asymmetry of the jaws more visible (Fig. 6.4).

The next step was to remove the lower splint and perform SARPE. Expansion started a week after surgery and was completed in a few weeks, achieving correction of the maxillary compression (Fig. 6.5).

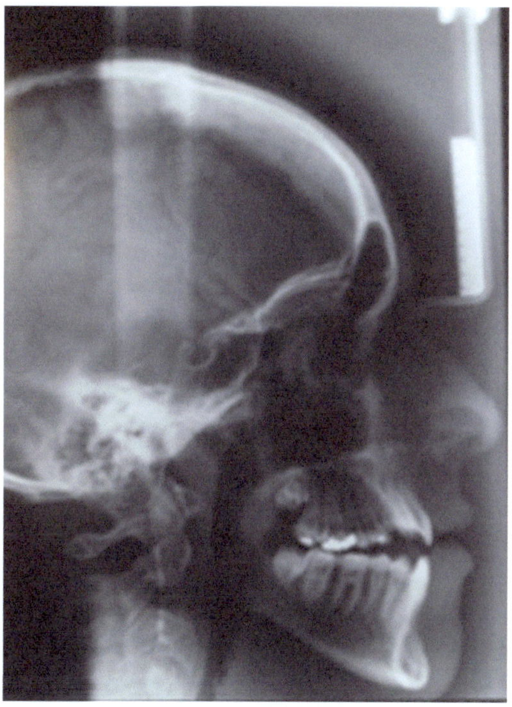

Fig. 6.3 Pretreatment teleradiographic view

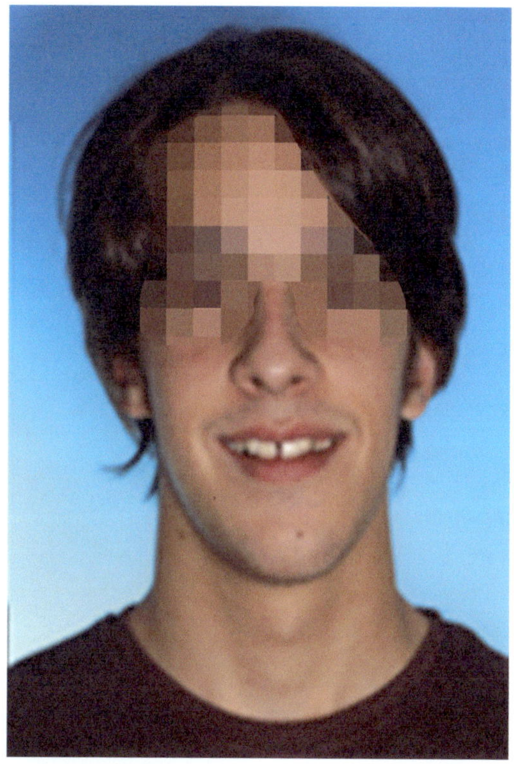

Fig. 6.5 Pre-SARPE teleradiographic (left) and intraoral photographic views (right)

Fig. 6.4 Pre-SARPE teleradiographic (left) and intraoral photographic views (right)

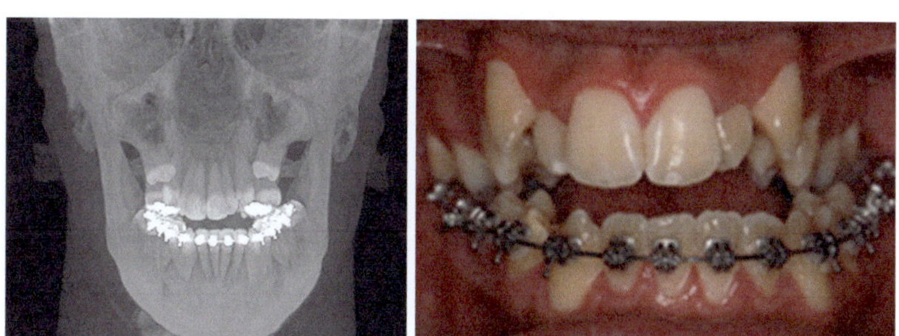

One month after the last round of expansion, we placed the upper brackets, and little by little, the interincisal diastema closed. In the following phase of orthodontics, the patient was prepared for orthognathic surgery for approximately 1 year. The dental arches were aligned and leveled to achieve class I occlusion once surgery was performed and the dental inclinations were normalized, so that they did not interfere with the skeletal movements necessary to correct the patient's occlusion and achieve improvement of the facial aesthetics (Figs. 6.6 and 6.7).

Once the patient was ready for surgery, no further movements were made to the teeth, and the necessary records were taken for surgical planning (facial and intraoral photos, intraoral scan, CBCT, and teleradiography) (Fig. 6.6, 6.7 and 6.8).

Preparation of the surgical guides was made with the 3D virtual design of surgery, superimposing the intraoral scanner and CBCT with Dolphin Imaging® (Fig. 6.9).

The scheduled surgery was bimaxillary, attempting a maxillary advancement of 8 mm, a mandibular advancement to achieve class I occlusion, with mandibular antero-rotation to close the

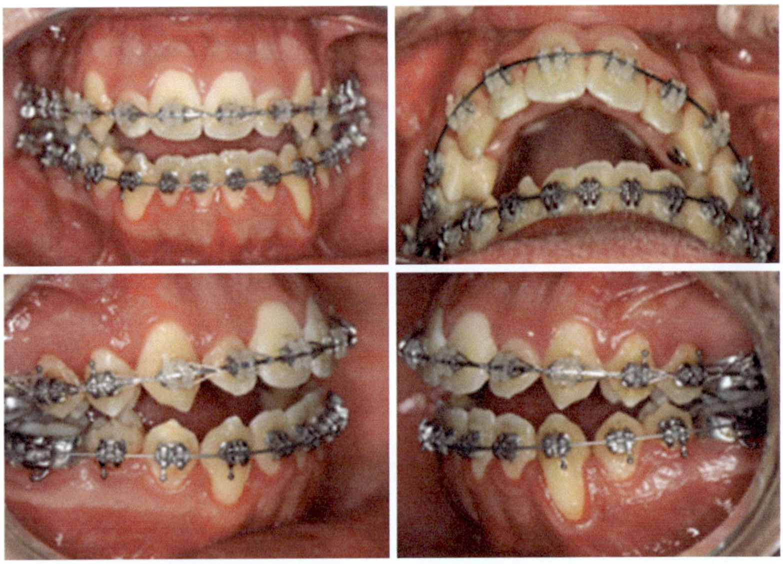

Fig. 6.6 Pre-orthognathic surgery intraoral views

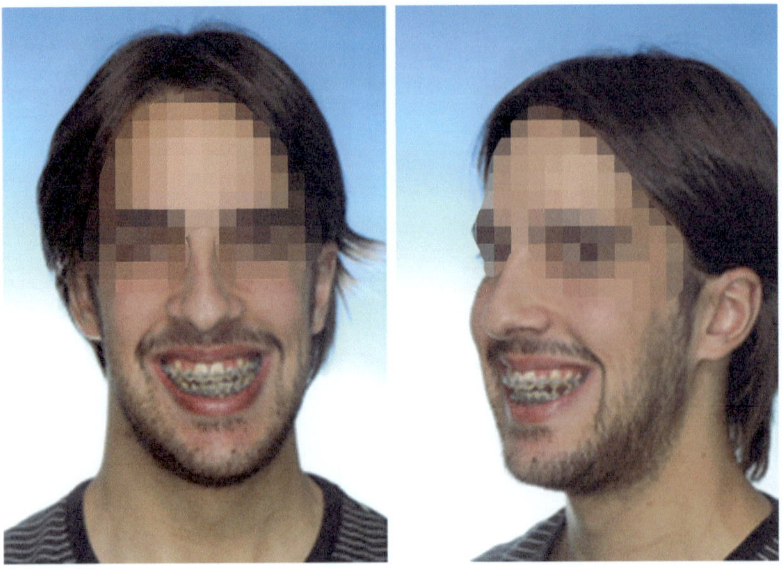

Fig. 6.7 Pre-orthognathic surgery extraoral views

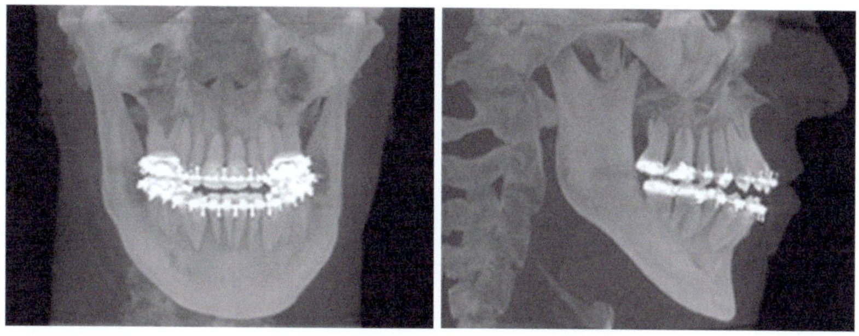

Fig. 6.8 Pre-orthognathic surgery CBCT scan

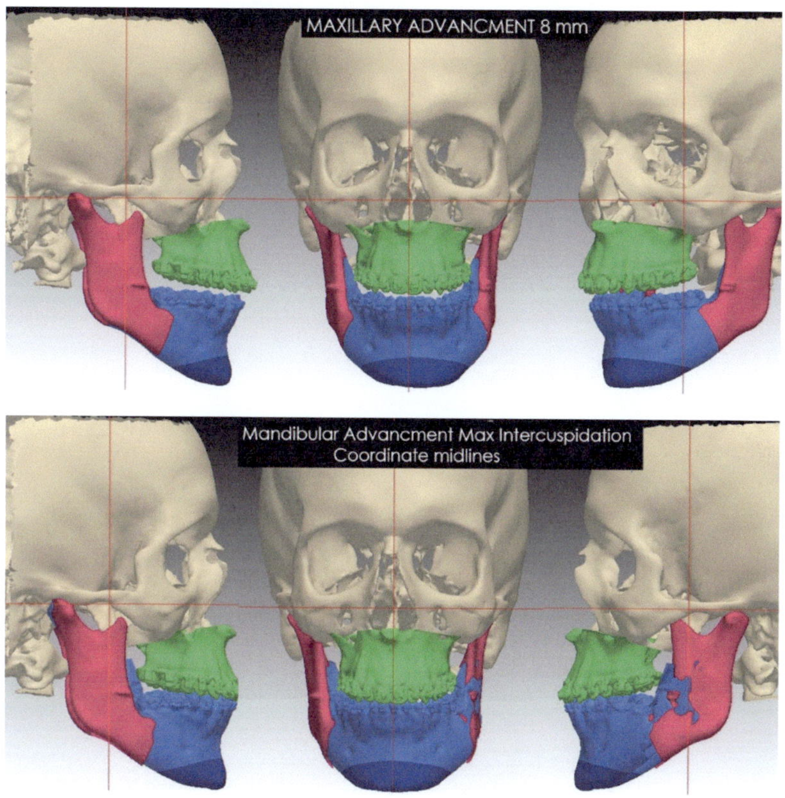

Fig. 6.9 Virtual surgical planning with Dolphin®

open bite and centering of the mandible to correct asymmetry.

One week after bimaxillary orthognathic surgery, we began to place intermaxillary elastics to improve the patient's occlusion.

The patient attended the orthodontic clinic 1 week after surgery to begin with occlusal control through intermaxillary elastics.

In the immediate postoperative period, acceptable occlusion, correction of asymmetry, and a correct overbite were achieved, but there was still some orthodontic time to improve all aspects of occlusion and the aesthetics of the patient's smile.

Little by little, the overbite, the dental fit, and the aesthetics of the smile were improved until the adequate aesthetic, occlusal, and functional objectives were achieved.

In the final images of the face, it can be seen how the width of the smile, the lateral projection, the mandibular asymmetry, and the smile arch have been improved (Fig. 6.10).

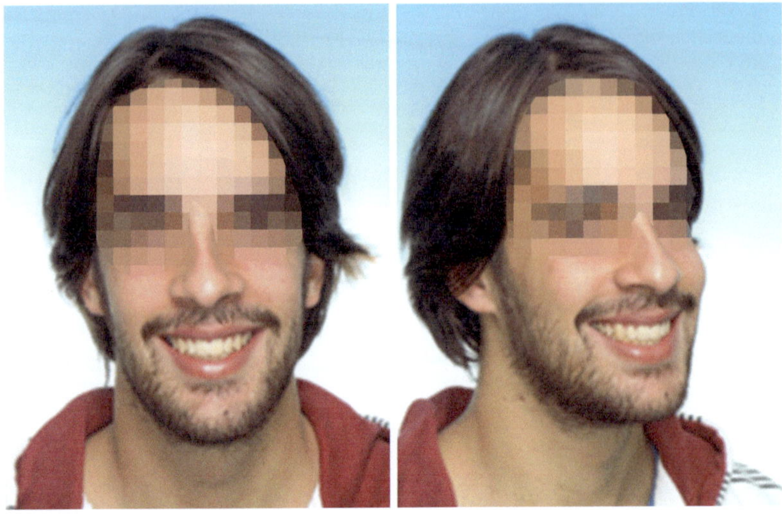

Fig. 6.10 Final treatment extraoral photographs

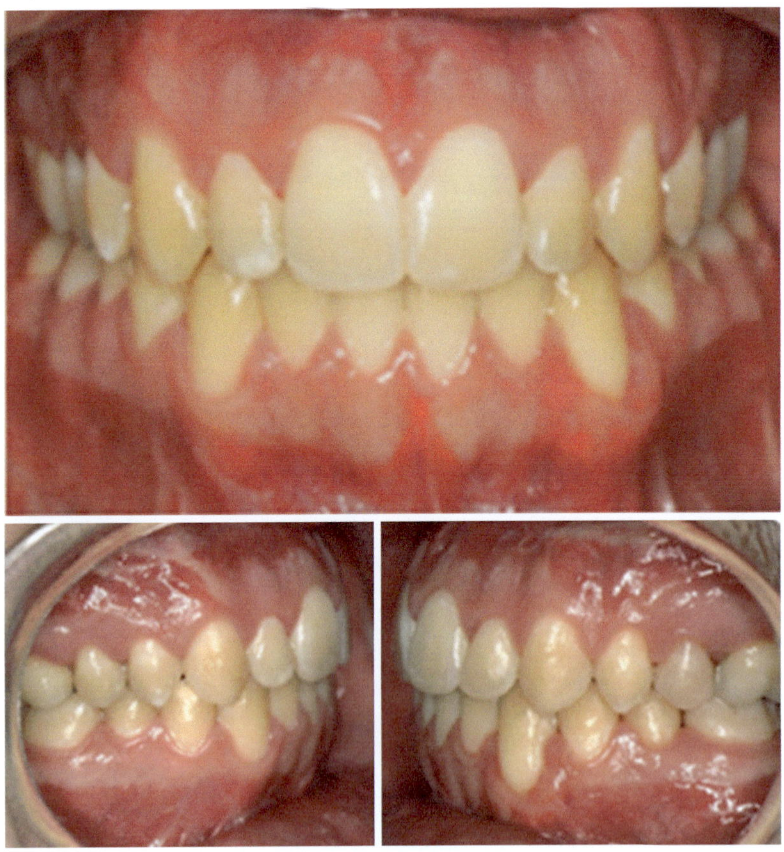

Fig. 6.11 Final treatment intraoral views

In the final intraoral images, we can see how the open bite has closed and how the dental occlusion and alignment of the teeth have improved, with adequate leveling of the gingival margins and the incisal edges (Fig. 6.11).

In the final teleradiographic, CBCT, and intraoral scan, adequate dental inclination, skeletal class I occlusion, and overbite can be observed, along with the titanium plates placed during surgery (Fig. 6.12).

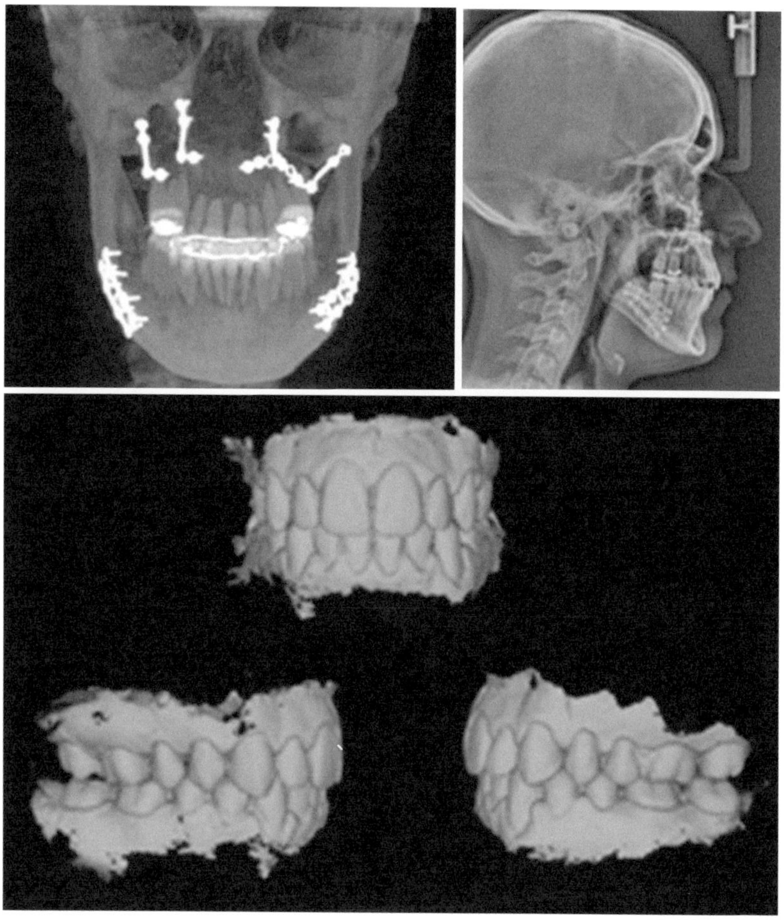

Fig. 6.12 Final treatment CBCT scan (top left), teleradiography (top right), and intraoral scan (below)

References

1. Lee K. Pre-orthodontic Orthognathic Surgery (POGS) using TADs: evidences and applications. Temporary skeletal anchorage devices. Berlin/Heidelberg: Springer; 2014. p. 209–29.
2. Shetye PR, Wirthlin JO. Orthodontist's role in orthognathic surgery. Semin Plast Surg. 2013;27(03):137.
3. Quast A, Santander P, Leding J, Klenke D, Moser N, Schliephake H, et al. Orthodontic incisor decompensation in orthognathic therapy—success and efficiency in three dimensions. Clin Oral Invest. 2020;25(6):4001–10.
4. Heda P, Raghuwanshi B, Prakash A, Sonawane K. Surgical orthodontics: literature review and case report. Int J Med Dent. 2013;3:38–46.
5. Hernández-Alfaro F, Guijarro-Martínez R. On a definition of the appropriate timing for surgical intervention in orthognathic surgery. Int J Oral Maxillofac Surg. 2014;43(7):846–55.
6. Sabri R. Orthodontic objectives in orthognathic surgery: state of the art today. World J Orthod. 2006;7(2):177–91.
7. Larson BE. Orthodontic preparation for orthognathic surgery. Oral Maxillofac Surg Clin North Am. 2014;26(4):441–58.
8. Park JH, Papademetriou M, Kwon Y. Orthodontic considerations in orthognathic surgery: who does what, when, where and how? Semin Orthod. 2016;22(1):2–11.
9. Jacobs SG. Treatment planning in orthodontics and orthognathic surgery: the significance of tooth inclination and dental compensations. Aust Dent J. 1991;36(5):349–55.
10. Hyun PJ. Temporary anchorage devices in clinical orthodontics. 1st ed. Hoboken: Wiley-Blackwell; 2020.
11. Yi J, Lu W, Xiao J, Li X, Li Y, Zhao Z. Effect of conventional combined orthodontic-surgical treatment on oral health-related quality of life: a systematic review and meta-analysis. Am J Orthod Dentofacial Orthop. 2019 Jul;156(1):29–43.e5.
12. Pérez Varela JC, Fonte A. Tratamiento del problema esquelético transversal en el paciente ortodóncico adulto.Ortodoncia española: Boletín de la Sociedad Española de. Ortodoncia. 2006;2:96–130.

13. Hernandez-Alfaro F. Upper incisor to Soft Tissue Plane (UI-STP): a new reference for diagnosis and planning in dentofacial deformities. Med Oral Patol Oral Cir Bucal. 2010;15(5):e779–81.
14. Klein KP, Kaban LB, Masoud MI. Orthognathic surgery and orthodontics. Oral Maxillofac Surg Clin North Am. 2020;32(1):71–82.
15. Wolford LM. Comprehensive post orthognathic surgery orthodontics. Oral Maxillofac Surg Clin North Am. 2020;32(1):135–51.

Clear Aligner Therapy in Orthognathic Surgery

7

Oriol Quevedo Pou, Fernando de la Iglesia Beyme, and Ariadna Pamies Parejo

7.1 Introduction

The aim of orthognathic surgery is to establish ideal dental occlusion between the maxilla and the mandible in order to optimize facial aesthetics, combining orthodontics and surgery. [1] Accordingly, orthognathic surgery has traditionally been linked to orthodontics with fixed appliances (dental braces) that are often regarded as an inconvenience by some patients. An alternative for these patients is the use of clear aligner therapy (CAT), which has become established as a novel option in orthognathic surgery [1] (Fig. 7.1).

However, some orthodontists may be reluctant to choose CAT when the treatment involves orthognathic surgery, due to difficulties in controlling the immediate postsurgical dental movement and postsurgical dental settling. Surprisingly, despite the popularity of clear aligners, the literature supporting the use of CAT in conjunction with orthognathic surgery mainly consists of case reports, in which multibracket appliances are often used at some point during orthodontic treatment and expert opinions on fixation methods and other techniques. [2–8]

In this chapter, we aim to provide a workflow involving the specialists—the orthodontist and surgeon—to secure a more predictable outcome when treating CAT patients who are scheduled for an orthofacial–orthognathic surgery procedure.

In hindsight, no one could have imagined the use of CAT in orthognathic surgery, though today it is a reality and a feasible option. Indeed, it can be affirmed that new approaches have defined CAT as the future of orthognathic surgery.

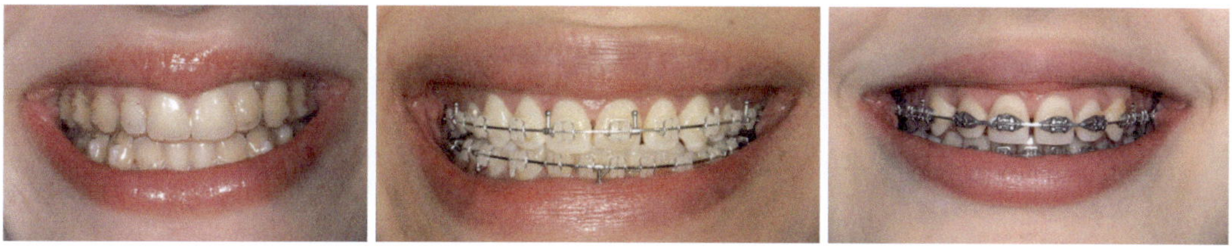

Fig. 7.1 Aesthetic appearance with the three most common orthodontic treatments. 1—Aligners, 2—Aesthetic braces, 3—Metallic braces

O. Quevedo Pou (✉) · F. de la Iglesia Beyme · A. Pamies Parejo
ORTODONCIA SANT CUGAT. Rambla del Celler 5, Sant Cugat del Vallès, Barcelona, Spain

F. Hernández-Alfaro, A. Valls Ontañón (eds.), *Orthofacial Surgery*,
https://doi.org/10.1007/978-3-031-76185-0_7

7.2 Presurgical Orthodontic Planning

Once records are obtained, including extra- and intraoral photos, a lateral cephalogram and panoramic radiographs—preferably but not necessarily cone-beam computed tomography (CBCT)—and an intraoral scan, the orthodontist prepares a preliminary virtual setup (usually called ClinCheck). The most important thing when performing this first three-dimensional (3D) plan is to know that the final 3D result obtained should not be the perfect one. This 3D plan must be the 3D plan of a decompensation, not that of a perfect dentition, and known as orthodontic surgical decompensation [8] (Fig. 7.2).

Often, the planned virtual movements are unrealistic or have low clinical predictability. [9] Therefore, for a more predictable outcome, an appropriate attachment design is needed, as well as improved staging of tooth movement. Additionally, overcorrection of certain movements, such as lower and upper incisor torque, is often planned. For this reason, if communication with the technician is problematic or it proves difficult to understand the decompensation process, we recommend using the 3D virtual controls to achieve the desired dental movements in this stage.

This digital treatment plan will estimate the decompensation movements based on our diagnosis. It is of paramount importance to consider the intra- and extraoral records in the virtual treatment plan. It should be noted that leveling and aligning of both arches should be achieved before surgery.

Outlined below are some of the more common aspects that should be considered during specific decompensation movements.

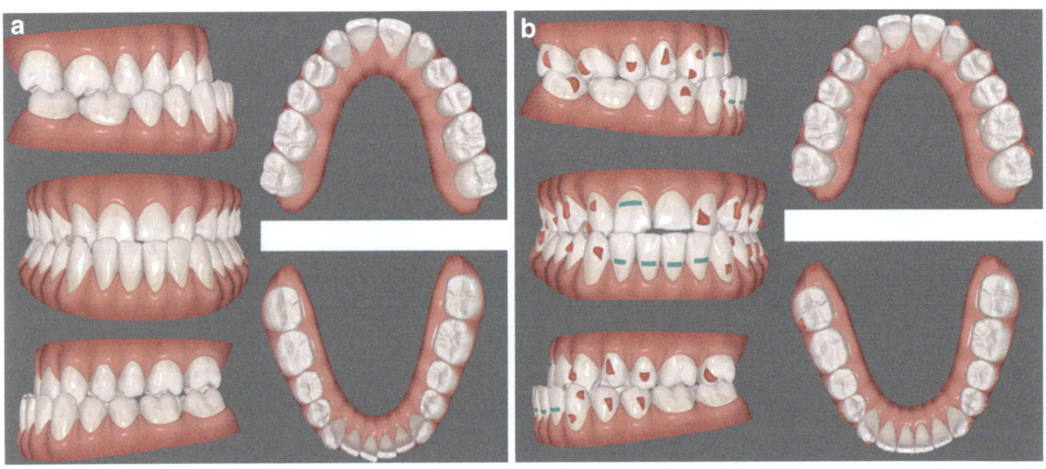

Fig. 7.2 Dental decompensation of class III malocclusion before surgery (**a**) Pretreatment, (**b**) Decompensation planned

7.3 Decompensation in Anteroposterior Discrepancies

The anteroposterior relationship and overjet ought to be worsened or, at least, left unchanged prior to surgery. For example, a skeletal class II malocclusion usually requires an increase in positive overjet, commonly achieved through proinclination of the upper incisors, retroinclination of the lower anterior teeth, or premolar extraction in the lower arch (Fig. 7.3). On the other hand, a skeletal class III malocclusion usually requires proinclination of the lower incisors to increase a negative overjet or premolar extraction in the upper arch (Fig. 7.4).

To achieve a more efficient virtual setup, Palone et al. [10] recommended an approximately 20.5% overcorrection in proinclination and retroinclination movements. Another recommended tool in the ClinCheck is visualization of the predicted Bolton analysis. The resolution of any Bolton discrepancy can facilitate decompensation via interproximal reduction and/or opening spaces to improve the probability of idealized occlusion during finishing and detailing [1] (Figs. 7.5 and 7.6).

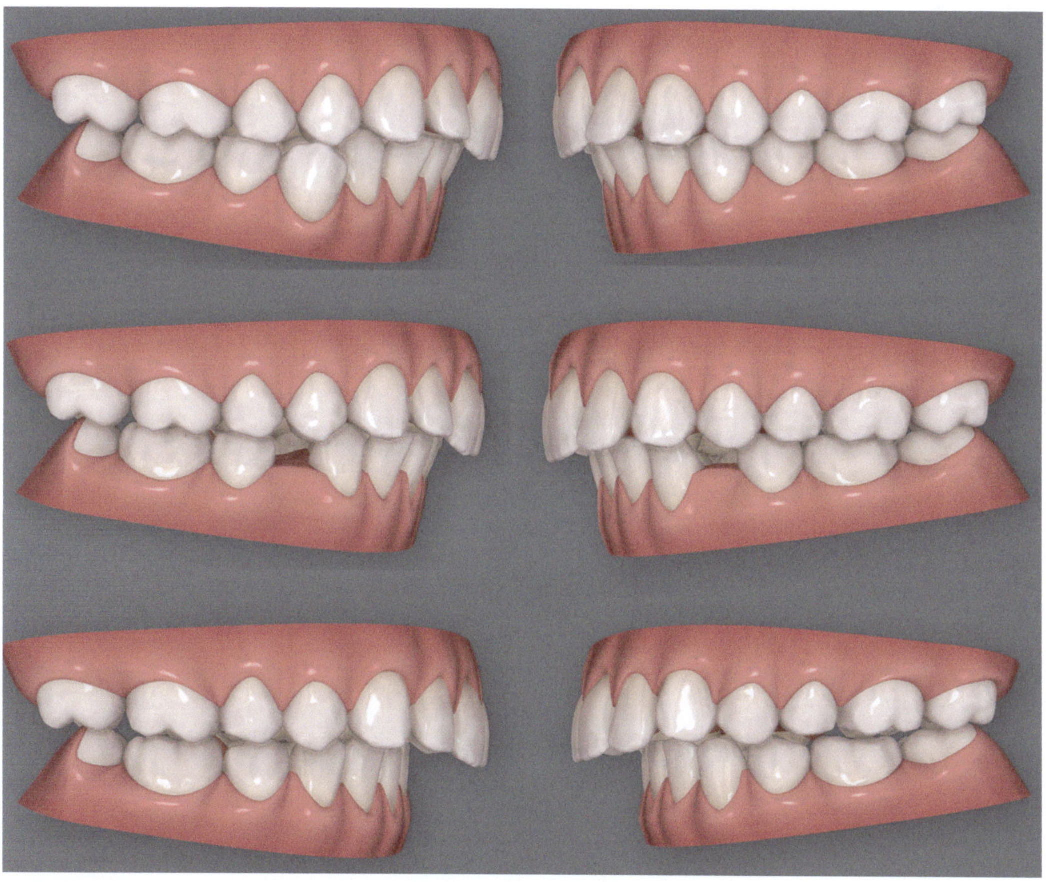

Fig. 7.3 Virtual setup of dental decompensation with lower premolar extraction of a skeletal class II patient being prepared for bimaxillary advancement treated with aligners

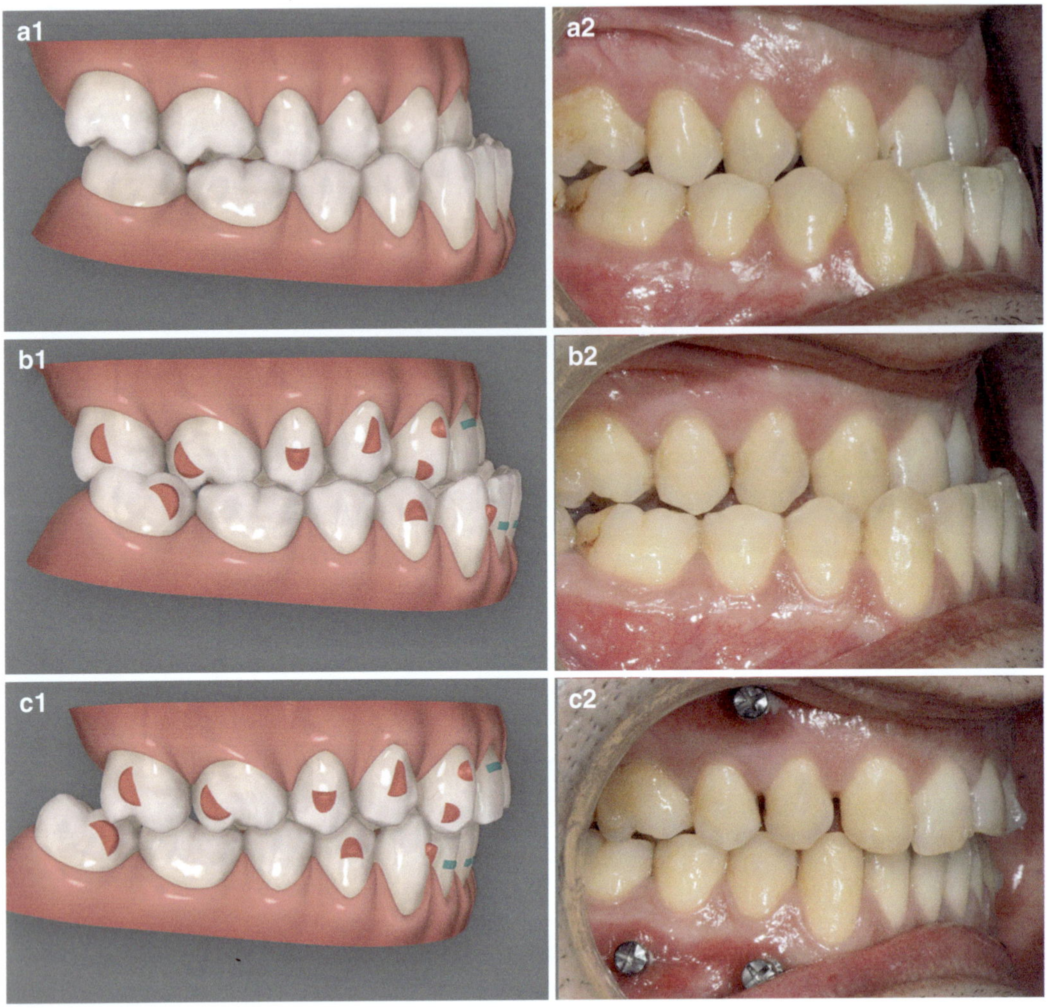

Fig. 7.4 A dental and skeletal class III patient treated with aligners and bimaxillary surgery. (**a**) Initial situation. (**b**) Dental decompensation. (**c**) Virtual jump and real surgery jump

Fig. 7.5 Dental situation of the decompensation process of the patient in Fig. 7.3 (**a**) Initial situation. (**b**) Dental extraction. (**c**) Dental decompensation. (**d**) Final occlusion after surgery and orthodontic refinement

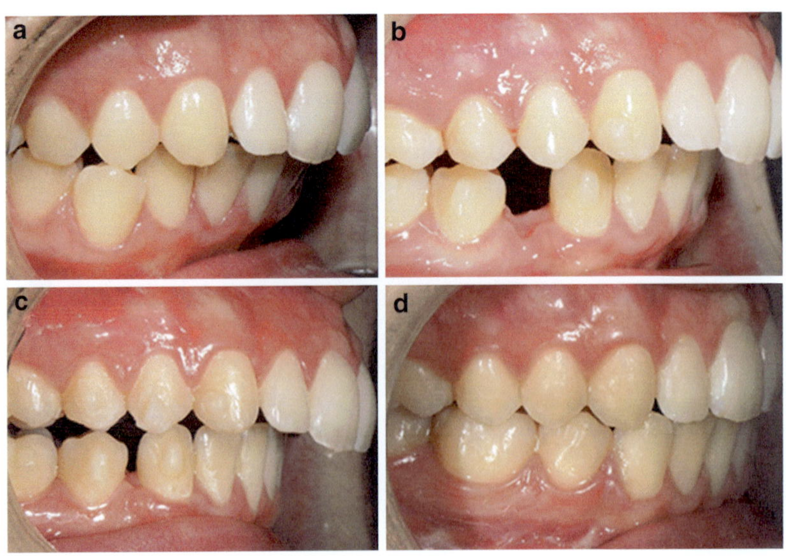

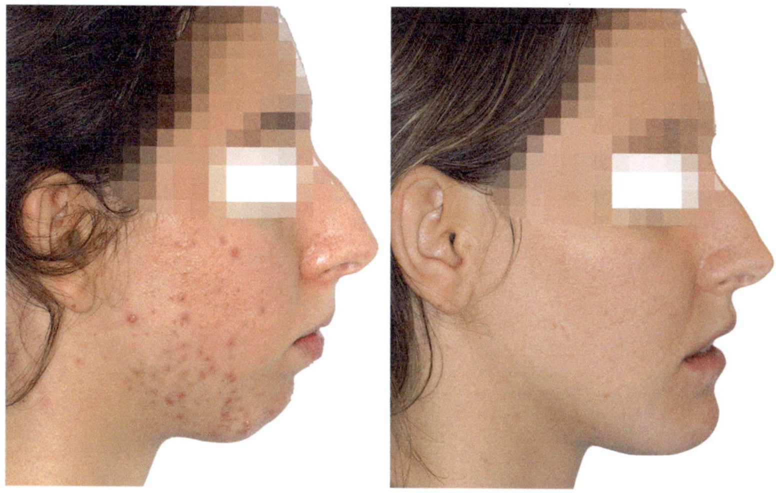

Fig. 7.6 Facial appearance before and after treatment corresponding to the patient in Fig. 7.3

7.4 Decompensation in Transverse Discrepancies

A patient with transverse discrepancy and posterior crossbite should not be corrected if the transverse discrepancy will be solved with segmental maxillary surgery. It is common to constrict the maxillary arch by correcting posterior molar buccolingual inclinations and to expand the mandibular arch to accentuate the transverse discrepancy in preparation for segmental surgery. In all these situations, the orthodontist when performing the 3D virtual plan should consider not only the crown position and inclination but also the root movement (Fig. 7.7).

If a three-piece maxillary surgery is to be performed, the orthodontist should open spaces for osteotomies distal to the maxillary lateral incisors and diverge the roots of both the canines and the lateral incisors. Hence, special attachments, such as twin attachments, are recommended for root movements. Moreover, a 14.5% overcorrection of tipping movement is recommended. [10]

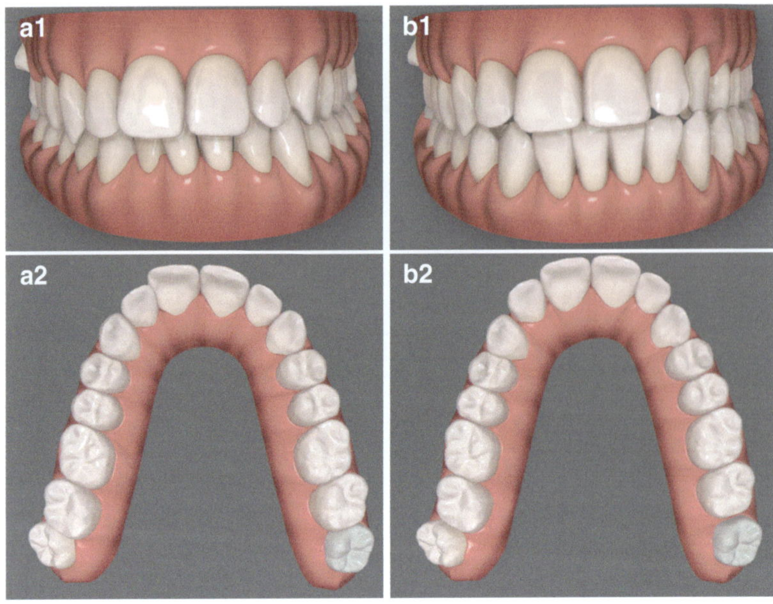

Fig. 7.7 Virtual decompensation in transverse discrepancy. Note that the crossbite is not corrected but rather increased and worsened. (**a**) Pretreatment, (**b**) Decompensation virtual planning

7.5 Decompensation in Vertical Discrepancies

When it comes to vertical dimension and overbite, the orthodontist should pay special attention to relapse. Tooth movements such as extrusion of the incisor in the anterior open bite malocclusion should be avoided. Preferably, the orthodontist should maintain the different planes during the decompensation, and leveling will be made with surgery (Fig. 7.8).

In deep bite malocclusions, tooth movements used to level the curve of Spee ought to be virtually overcorrected due to a lack of full clinical expression of movements that rely on attachments (horizontal or retentive type [11]) in the anterior and posterior segments.

In addition to the attachments, bite ramps in the aligners can be prescribed to help in the correction of deep bite malocclusions. [12]

In contrast, patients with skeletal class II division 2 malocclusion and a short face should have the curve of Spee corrected postsurgically in order to increase the anterior facial height. [13] With this approach, it is important to maintain dental tripodism before surgery and just after surgery, as premolars will be extruded in the postsurgical phase with CAT (Fig. 7.9).

Specifically, extrusion of the posterior teeth and intrusion of the anterior teeth, resulting in overcorrection to a simulated open bite, should be incorporated to the digital plan. Attachments should be placed in molars and premolars, and horizontal beveled attachments (HBAs) are the preferred option on the mandibular canines. All these steps required in the virtual treatment software should be used as a visual representation of forces rather than as a predictor of final tooth position [11] (Fig. 7.10, 7.11, and 7.12).

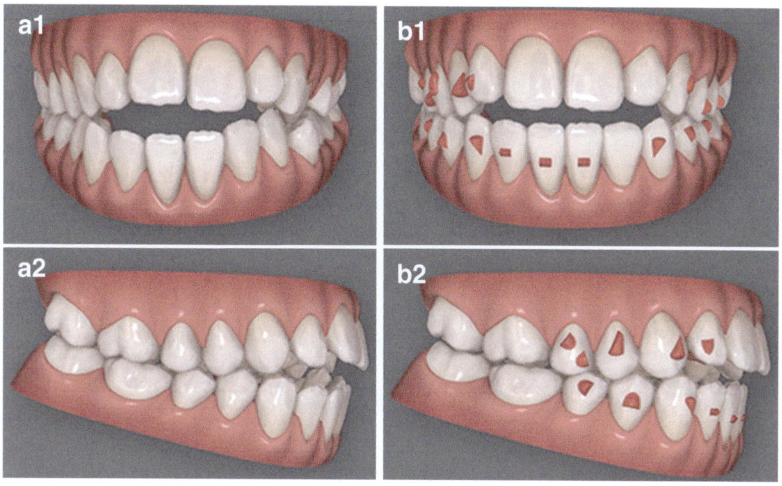

Fig. 7.8 Virtual decompensation in vertical discrepancy. Note that the double occlusal plan is maintained. This should be corrected by the surgeon. (**a**) Pretreatment, (**b**) Decompensation virtual planning

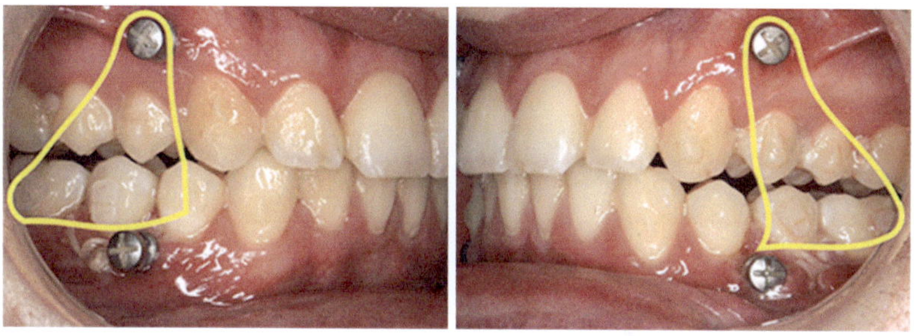

Fig. 7.9 Use of elastics after surgery in a short face patient to correct the curve of Spee. From TADs to dental buttons

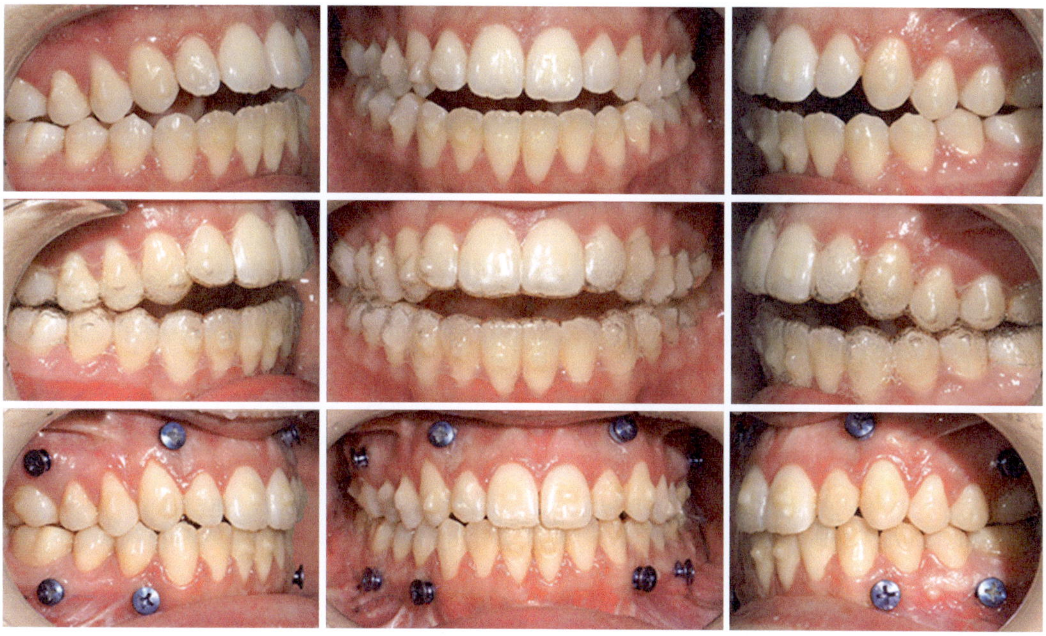

Fig. 7.10 Follow-up of the patient in Fig. 7.8. Dental follow-up

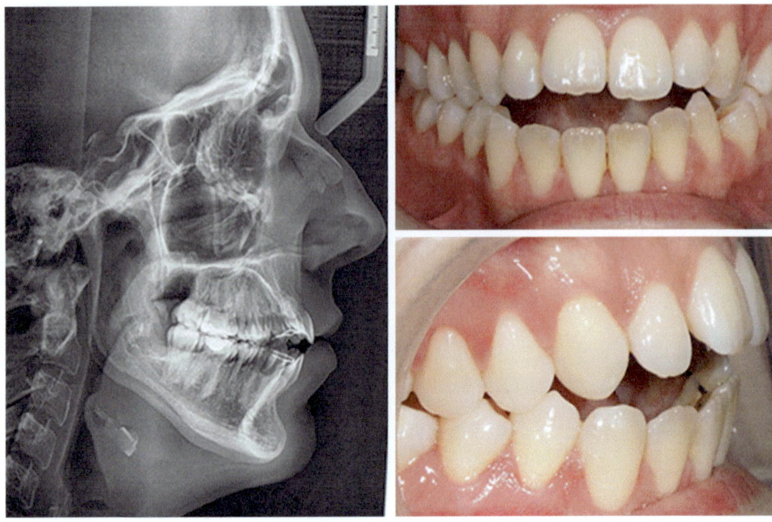

Fig. 7.11 Initial situation of the patient in Fig. 7.8

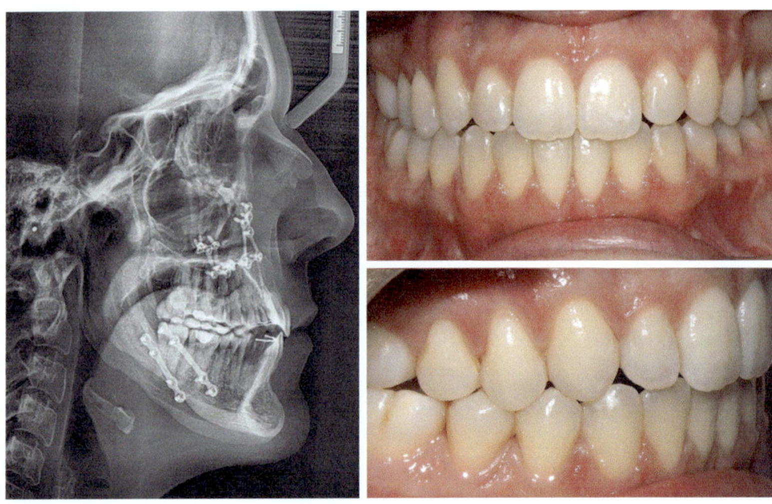

Fig. 7.12 Final situation of the patient in Fig. 7.8

7.6 Decompensation in Dentofacial Asymmetry

In most cases, skeletal asymmetry leads to midline deviations. Midline discrepancies in bimaxillary surgeries should be left untouched or even worsened in the presurgical phase, whereas in single-jaw surgeries, midline orthodontic correction should only be performed in the non-affected arch, which is often the maxilla.

Once decompensation movements have been virtually planned in the virtual 3D plan, virtual surgery (bite jump or virtual jump) follows as the last step in the setup. It comprises a single stage of immediate arch coordination simulating the surgical outcome, after orthodontic decompensation movements, allowing both arches to occlude in class I. This should be exclusively performed by the technician (Fig. 7.13).

Once the digital treatment plan has been developed, both professionals review it to make sure mutual goals are achieved, as coordination is the key, as outlined by others. [2] The final digital treatment plan is then accepted and sent for aligner fabrication. The patient will begin the orthodontic treatment with aligners, wearing them an average of 20–22 h per day.

When proper decompensation has been achieved, another virtual surgical planning is performed to allow confirmation of the surgical

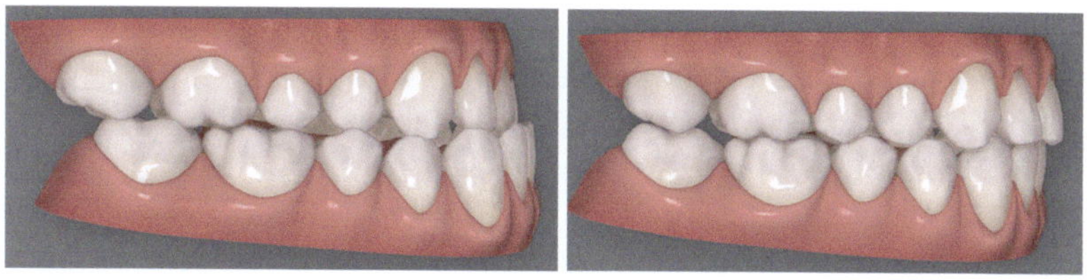

Fig. 7.13 Virtual bite jump made by the technician

movements without occlusal interferences. If the presurgical decompensation movements are achieved, the planning and fabrication of surgical splints can be initiated. At this point, the patient must wear a passive aligner to avoid any additional dental movements. By combining digital scanning for aligners with computer-aided surgical simulation, the surgical splint fabrication process is simplified.

In sum, an accurate workflow is detailed below:

1. First patient visit to the orthodontist or surgeon: Depending on the chief complaint of the patient, he/she will visit one of these specialists. Ideally, this visit would be with both members of the team.
2. Orthodontist: Full photographic records, a lateral and panoramic radiograph, an intraoral scan, and optionally a CBCT scan for the orthodontic diagnosis and treatment plan are needed.
3. Meeting between surgeon and orthodontist: Analysis and study are made of the surgical treatment objectives (STOs) for the orthognathic surgery patient with designing of a virtual surgical plan (VSP).
4. Starting orthodontic treatment: This involves dental decompensation as planned meticulously.

Once dental decompensation has been achieved and the patient wears passive aligners.

5. Surgeon: The patient visits the maxillofacial surgeon, and new records are taken—a set of photos, intraoral scans, a record of centric relation, and radiographs.
6. Meeting between surgeon and orthodontist: Another meeting is necessary in order to verify the surgical movements with another virtual surgical plan (VSP). The aim of this meeting is to make sure that all the presurgical tooth movements meet the requirements of the surgeon for adequate postsurgical occlusion. If this is not the case, refinement focused on the specific dental movements required by the surgeon will be necessary.
7. Surgeon: Designing and fabrication of the surgical splints. Once the splints are ready, the surgeon must try them on the patient to ensure perfect adjustment except in those patients who undergo maxilla segmentation, as the splints will not fit in.
8. Orthodontist: Scanning is made of the upper and the lower arch with all the attachments, without the occlusion scan. A detailed explanation of this will be given later in the "Postsurgical Orthodontic Considerations" section.
9. Surgery day with the surgeon: The patient should wear the aligners all the day and remove them 20 min before surgery.

Cong et al. [14] concluded that clear aligners can be considered for presurgical orthodontics; tooth movements involved in arch leveling and decompensations are seen to be highly accurate when comparing the simulated and the clinically achieved movements.

7.7 Orthodontic Considerations During Surgery

The most common reasons why clear aligners and surgery have been considered incompatible are control of the osteotomized segments, fixation of the dentoalveolar complex and dental arches during surgery, and the inability to scan the arches because the patient cannot open the mouth properly until the fourth to fifth week after surgery. In our experience, temporary skeletal anchorage devices (TADs) are the ideal option, as has been the surgical approach with lingual appliances. [15]

Regarding the placement procedure, TADs are placed in each quadrant to be used for intermaxillary fixation during surgery. Usually, two TADs are placed in each quadrant, one between the canine and the first premolar (or between the first and second premolars), and another between the second premolar and first molar. We do not recommend using TADs in the anterior area (mesial to the canines) because of the increased risk of discomfort to the patient caused by gingival irritation.

When TADs are placed, there are various elastic choices depending on the initial malocclusion involved: the surgical patient will wear vertical elastics (1/8 6 oz) if the initial malocclusion was skeletal class I; class III elastics (3/16 4 oz) if it was skeletal class III; and class II elastics (3/16 4 oz) if it was skeletal class II before surgery. In dentofacial asymmetries, we recommend employing vertical elastics.

7.8 Segmental Surgery Considerations

When segmental expansion of the maxillary arch is performed, we recommend a technique that consists of using a palatal acrylic Hawley expander fixed to two TADs without tooth contact, which is placed during surgery (Fig. 7.14).

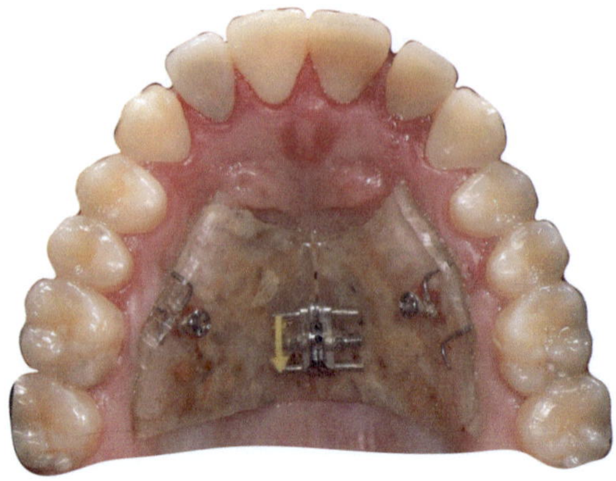

Fig. 7.14 Hawley expander appliance with no dental contact fixed to the palate with two mini-screws

The key aspect is to ensure bone stability and prevent bony segments from moving while simultaneously allowing tooth movement. During surgery, the surgeon stabilizes the Hawley expander with Adams hooks attached to the molars or premolars. A few days after surgery, when the patient reports to the orthodontist, the hooks are cut or maintained, depending on the postsurgical stability achieved. This method allows us to prescribe more expansion turns in the event of some transverse relapse. To ensure the stability of the expansion, the patient must wear the splint between 4 and 8 weeks, depending on his/her discomfort with the device. However, as this palatal Hawley expander does not have dental contacts, it is feasible to continue moving teeth normally without waiting for the healing of the bone to occur in order to start upper arch dental movements.

A similar clinical recommendation to maintain the transverse dimension achieved after surgery is to prescribe four passive aligners when maxillary cast segmentation in the VSP is performed. Thus, if surgery goes as planned in the cast surgery, the patient will be able to wear the new aligners, maintaining the stability of the maxillary segmentation. Nevertheless, there are certain limitations with this approach. Because not all surgical outcomes match the virtual plan, the aligner may not fit in the arch as desired; therefore, a palatal acrylic Hawley expander with two TADs is more effective in maintaining transverse dimension compared with aligners.

7.9 Postsurgical Considerations

After surgery, the patient is requested to wear the passive aligners as soon as possible. This may depend on the postsurgical recovery, since some patients can start wearing the aligners after 48 h, while others do so after 1 week. Nonetheless, it is essential to apply full-time TAD-to-TAD elastics at least during the first month.

The patient visits the orthodontist the first 1–2 weeks after surgery to confirm the correct use of the elastics and to scan both sides of the occlusion using the last upper and lower arches obtained a few days before surgery. As a result of this, it is possible to send new records for a new ClinCheck for new detailing, consequently saving time as otherwise the upper and lower arches would not be able to be scanned for at least a month because of the inability of the patient to open the mouth. However, this method is largely unpredictable and inaccurate in the segmental surgery of the maxillary arch, due to arch form changes. [1] Therefore, in some cases, it is necessary to scan the patient 4–6 weeks after surgery to obtain refinement aligners for these patients.

Postsurgical elastics are frequently essential to maintain and support the corrected occlusion; a variation of elastics may be needed during monitoring. The elastics can be attached to the orthodontic TADs, to orthodontic buttons, or also to aligner notches. In some scenarios, such as in patients with skeletal class II malocclusion and short face patterns, it is preferable to correct the curve of Spee postsurgically. In this case, it is preferable to place buttons in the lower premolars bonded gingivally and to attach an elastic extending from the upper TAD to the lower premolars. Thus, the curve of Spee is corrected by premolar extrusion more quickly and efficiently, with appropriate patient compliance.

Additionally, in cases where settling of posterior buccal segments is required, the aligner can be cut posteriorly to secure better and stable occlusion.

7.10 Surgery First

The surgery first (SF) approach in orthognathic surgery is popular among patients due to the immediate improvement of the facial profile it affords. Some authors [7] have already published case reports with clear aligner therapy and SF.

It should be taken into account that SF demands more precise orthognathic surgery. Radiographs and intraoral–extraoral records are necessary, as well as VSP and STOs. Furthermore, the patient should be scanned before surgery.

With all these records, a virtual jump in the ClinCheck is planned together with the surgeon. Once the virtual jump is done, the correction of dental alterations such as crowding is prescribed. Next, the patient undergoes surgery, in which the surgeon must be extremely precise in order for the aligners to fit perfectly, since the surgical splints have been designed according to the virtual jump of the digital planning. The surgeon also places several TADs during surgery, and the patient will wear TAD-to-TAD elastics immediately after surgery in conjunction with the aligners.

Unfortunately, there are cases in which the aligners do not fit in after surgery. It is in these patients where a full new scan of the arches with the postsurgical occlusion is required in order to determine a new plan in the ClinCheck. In contrast to the ideal SF planning previously described, if this protocol is followed, it will take approximately three more weeks for the aligners to be manufactured, so the patient will be free of appliances during this entire period.

7.11 Conclusions

In conclusion, CAT for orthognathic surgery is becoming a daily routine. The paradigm has shifted completely in both the orthodontic approach and in intraoperative management. However, several technical and biomechanical factors must be considered, and adequate professional experience (on the part of the surgeon and orthodontist) is required, in the same way as good communication between them throughout the treatment.

References

1. Moshiri M. Considerations for treatment of patients undergoing orthognathic surgery using clear aligners. AJO-DO Clin Companion. 2022;2:1–11.
2. Taub DI, Palermo V. Orthognathic surgery for the Invisalign patient. Semin Orthod. 2017;23(1):99–102.
3. Aziz SR. Clear aligner orthognathic surgery: a narrative review. Front Oral Maxillofac Med. 2021:1–5.
4. Pagani R, Signorino F, Poli PP, Manzini P, Panisi I. The use of invisalign® system in the management of the orthodontic treatment before and after Class III surgical approach. Case Rep Dent. 2016;2016:1–11.

5. Lin JCY, Chen S, Liou EJW, Ojima K, Bowman SJ. Interdisciplinary aligner treatment of short-face patients. JCO. 2017;LI(7):382–405.
6. Zhang W, Yang H. Orthognathic surgery in invisalign patients. J Craniofac Surg. 2022;33(2):E112–3.
7. Kook MS, Kim HM, Oh HK, Lee KM. Clear aligner use following surgery-first mandibular prognathism correction. J Craniofac Surg. 2019;30(6):e544–7.
8. Lou T, Caminiti M. Orthognathic surgery combined with clear aligner therapy. JCO. 2021;LV(1):44–58.
9. Al-Nadawi M, Kravitz ND, Hansa I, Makki L, Ferguson DJ, Vaid NR. Effect of clear aligner wear protocol on the efficacy of tooth movement: a randomized clinical trial. Angle Orthod. 2021;91(2):157–63.
10. Palone M, Pignotti A, Morin E, Pancari C, Spedicato GA, Cremonini F, et al. Analysis of overcorrection to be included for planning clear aligner therapy: a retrospective study. Angle Orthod. 2022;00(00):1–8.
11. Kravitz ND, Moshiri M, Nicozisis J, Miller S. Mechanical considerations for deep-bite correction with aligners. Semin Orthod. 2020;26(3):134–8.
12. Khosravi R, Cohanim B, Hujoel P, Daher S, Neal M, Liu W, et al. Management of overbite with the Invisalign appliance. Am J Orthod Dentofacial Orthop. 2017;151(4):691–9.
13. Sabri R. Orthodontic objectives in orthognathic surgery: historical development. World J Orthod. 2006;7(2):177–91.
14. Cong A, Ruellas AC d O, Tai SK, Loh CT, Barkley M, Yatabe M, et al. Presurgical orthodontic decompensation with clear aligners. Am J Orthod Dentofacial Orthop. 2022;162(4):538–53.
15. De la Iglesia F, Pinós H, Arcas A, Wallter A, Clusellas N, De la Iglesia G, et al. Bimaxillary surgery with maxillary segmentation and lingual orthodontics. EC Dent Sci. 2018;17(1):7–14.

8 Three-Dimensional Planning in Orthofacial Surgery

Orion-Luiz Haas-Junior

The current state of orthognathic surgery, referred to as contemporary orthognathic surgery, has promoted shifts in paradigms over the years (Fig. 8.1). Among these shifts, virtual planning has elevated the conventional treatment model to a three-dimensional (3D) environment, allowing greater assertiveness during surgical procedures, and has become an invaluable tool in the diagnosis of dentofacial deformities. Another major paradigm shift is the adoption of an orthofacial surgery mentality for clinical diagnosis and surgical treatment. This new approach to the treatment of dentofacial deformities has enabled surgical planning and treatment not only of dental occlusions but also of additional functional and aesthetic complaints reported by patients.

Virtual planning has helped surgeons to develop their skills beyond the treatment of dental occlusion, identify other functional problems such as upper airway obstruction due to dentofacial deformities, and pay more consideration to facial aesthetics. This is possible thanks to more precise surgical procedures resulting from the visualization, in a single image, of bone structures, dental occlusions, temporomandibular joints, soft tissue face mask, and the airway (Fig. 8.2).

The combination of 3D tools with an orthofacial mentality at the time of diagnosis and during surgical procedures in the treatment of dentofacial deformities is the most important paradigm shift in recent years. This current symbiosis between a virtual environment (3D planning) and clinical diagnosis (orthofacial surgery) is the topic we aim to discuss in this chapter.

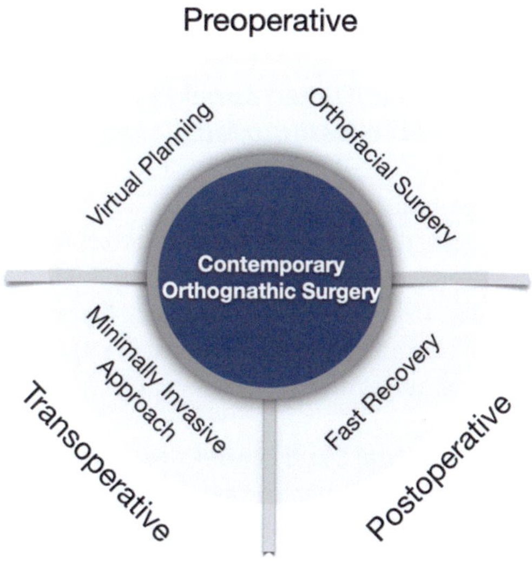

Fig. 8.1 Contemporary orthognathic surgery, new approaches in treatment stages

O.-L. Haas-Junior (✉)
Department of Oral and Maxillofacial Surgery, Hospital São Lucas – Pontifícia Universidade Católica do Rio Grande do Sul, Porto Alegre, Brazil

Blanc Hospital, Porto Alegre, Brazil

F. Hernández-Alfaro, A. Valls Ontañón (eds.), *Orthofacial Surgery*,
https://doi.org/10.1007/978-3-031-76185-0_8

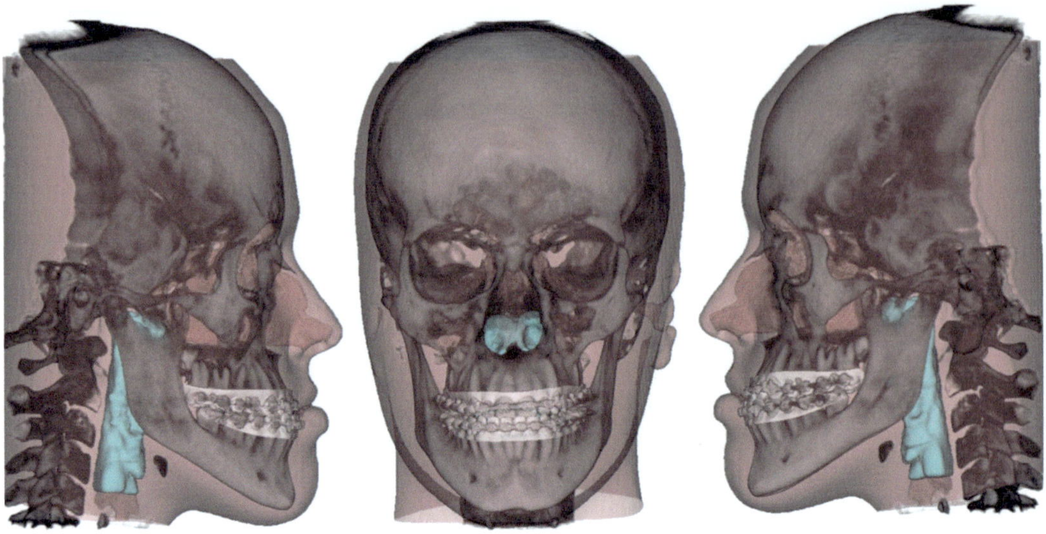

Fig. 8.2 Virtual skull model

8.1 Three-Dimensional Planning

The virtual planning protocol we use is based on simple steps that facilitate its application in non-academic settings (e.g., private practice) as much as possible while stressing a rigorous acquisition of photographs, computed tomography (CT) scans, and intraoral scans.

8.1.1 Three-Dimensional Planning of the *Instituto Maxilofacial*

Data acquisition for 3D surgical planning takes place a few days before surgery to warrant that no dental movements are expected beyond this moment. Because of this, in surgery-first cases, we want the arches to be placed just (24 h) before the actual surgery.

8.1.1.1 Virtual Skull Model Creation

A cone-beam computed tomography (CBCT) scan is taken with the radiological parameters set to 120 kV, 5 mA, scan time 7 s. The axial slice distance for each scan is 0.300 mm^3. A 23 cm field of view (FOV) is used. The patient is oriented breathing quietly, sitting upright in the natural head position (NHP), with the tongue in a relaxed position, and with the mandible in centric relation. Primary images are stored as 576 DICOM data files. The DICOM files are imported to Dolphin 3D Imaging software (Dolphin Imaging & Management Solutions, Chatsworth, CA, USA) in order to obtain a virtual skull model for surgical planning.

On the same day the patient undergoes the CBCT scan, surface scanning of both dental arches is performed with an intraoral scanner, thus producing an STL file. Then, the intraoral scanner of the dental occlusion (STL files) is superimposed over the dental occlusion area of the CBCT image (DICOM files) using a "best fit" algorithm. A soft-tissue facemask and the upper airway volume are also generated through the CBCT dataset. Pictures or 3D face scans of the patient can be incorporated to the 3D skeleton. The virtual skull model is thus generated (Fig. 8.2).

At this point, we perform the most important and sensitive part of 3D planning: 3D head orientation of the virtual patient. Frontal and lateral pictures of the patient taken in the NHP are used for this purpose. Needless to say, it is important to spend enough time taking those pictures and making sure they correspond to a reproducible NHP [1] (Fig. 8.3).

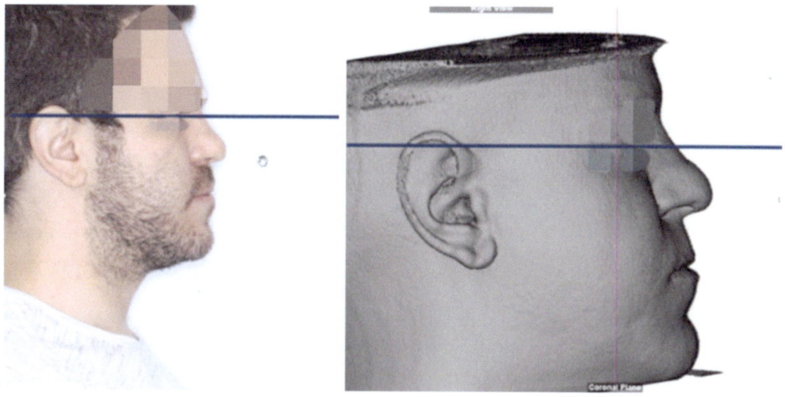

Fig. 8.3 NHP with photos. Blue line must be reproduced by NHP photo to 3D soft-tissue mask in virtual planning software

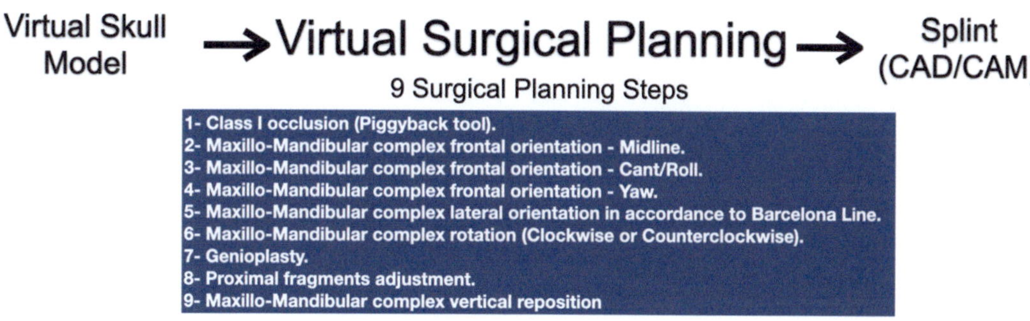

Fig. 8.4 *Instituto Maxilofacial* protocol; virtual surgical planning steps

8.1.1.2 Virtual Surgical Planning Steps

Physical cast models of both arches are placed in the ideal anticipated final occlusion and optically scanned. The STL file generated is then exported to the software, and with the "piggyback tool," the mandible is automatically moved into class I with the maxilla. This is the first virtual skeletal movement performed.

In the *Instituto Maxilofacial* protocol, the 3D planning sequence and steps are as follows (Fig. 8.4):

1. Mandible goes to the anticipated class I occlusion, mimicking the one previously set with cast models and transformed after scanning into an STL file.
2. Placing of horizontal and vertical gridlines.
3. Bimaxillary repositioning of the maxillo-mandibular complex (MMC) in the frontal plane.
   3a. Matching between dental and facial midlines.
   3b. Cant correction, using horizontal and vertical gridlines as reference. This includes cant correction of the chin in the event genioplasty is anticipated.
   3c. Yaw correction, using horizontal and vertical gridlines as reference. This includes yaw correction of the chin in the event genioplasty is anticipated.
4. Turning of the virtual patient to visualize the right lateral profile and place gridlines.
5. Moving one of the vertical lines at the soft-tissue nasion. This will be the soft-tissue plane or Barcelona Line [2] (Fig. 8.5a).
6. Displacement of the MMC until the edge of the upper incisor reaches the Barcelona Line (Fig. 8.5b).
7. Moving the center of rotation of the complex to some anatomical landmark such as the incisal edge, anterior nasal spine, posterior nasal spine, or pogonion.
8. If a genioplasty has been designed, movement of the chin to the appropriate position

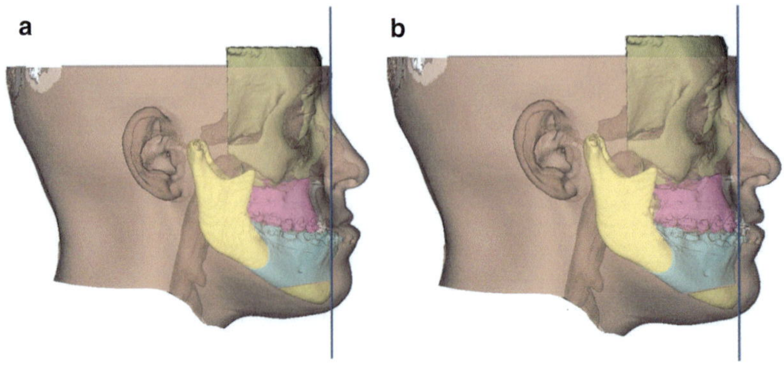

Fig. 8.5 (**a**) Barcelona Line as an anteroposterior reference prior to surgical movement. (**b**) Barcelona Line as an anteroposterior reference after surgical movement

(90° with respect to the mandibular occlusal plane).

9. Application of the necessary rotational movements of the MMC to achieve adequate projection of pogonion and paranasal areas (counterclockwise or clockwise).
10. In the case of a big step at the level of mandibular osteotomy, rotation of the posterior fragments accordingly to reduce/soften this step.
11. Adjustment of the vertical MMC position in accordance with the relation between the upper lip and upper incisors.
12. Adaption of the posterior (condylar) fragments to achieve symmetry and identify possible collision points between these fragments and the lingula on the proximal fragments.
13. Selection between mandible and maxilla first options. We usually select mandible first.
14. Printing of the intermediate and final splint.

By no means should the 3D planning software tell us where to reposition the MMC. Instead, we transfer our orthofacial-oriented plan into the 3D environment and warrant through the splints that this plan matches the actual surgical procedure [3, 4]. In other words, our orthofacial mentality rules the virtual surgical planning and not the other way around.

Construction of the virtual skull model by superimposing CBCT, scanned dental arches, and pictures takes roughly 30 min. Orienting the head of the patient, performing the osteotomies, and repositioning the MMC must be done by the surgeon and takes 15 min in standard cases and up to 30 min in complex asymmetric cases.

Previous publications on this protocol have shown that this is not only user-friendly but also accurate—with errors of less than 1 mm (0.1–0.9 mm) [3–5].

8.2 Three-Dimensional Planning and Soft-Tissue Aesthetics

Cone-beam computed tomography allows the creation of a facial mask by transforming the soft-tissue DICOM files into STL files (Fig. 8.6), which helps us diagnose deformities such as asymmetric or thin lips, nasal asymmetries, and an excess of submental tissues. We can then correlate these soft-tissue changes with bone structures to diagnose whether orthofacial surgery will help correct the deformity.

In relation to soft tissue simulation, the current software is not exact and can only be "approximative" at best. The reason for this is the enormous variability in soft-tissue quality among individuals and the lack of data regarding its reaction to complex skeletal movements. This makes it very difficult for an algorithm to accurately interpret reactions at the facial mask level [5, 6]. Hence, most software applications offer the possibility to subjectively modify the final soft-tissue profile according to the experience of the surgeon in a rather "artistic" way.

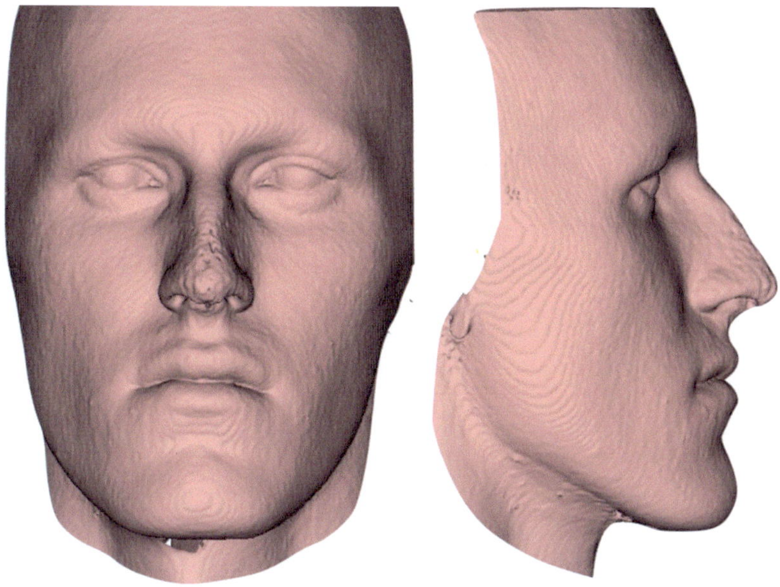

Fig. 8.6 Soft tissue mask

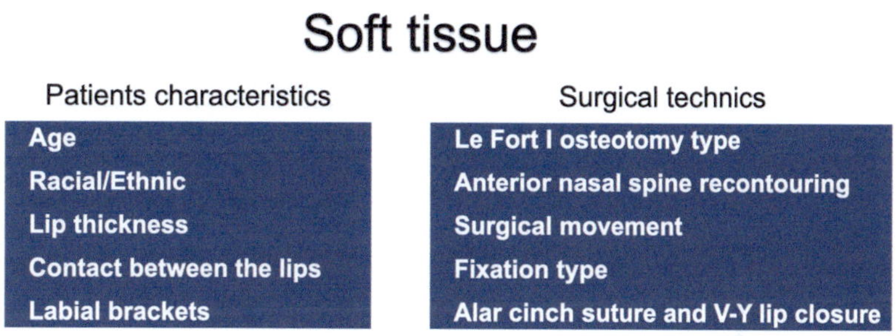

Fig. 8.7 Patient characteristics and surgical techniques

Patients frequently want to see the simulation of the 3D planning. It is always important to tell them that this simulation is only approximative and reflects the "direction" of the anticipated change—not the actual final result. It is already known that the use of 3D soft tissue tools to help communication between surgeon and patient brings more satisfaction to the patient during treatment [7].

8.2.1 Soft Tissue Simulation: "Approximative" at Best

As previously mentioned, soft-tissue response to the surgical movement of bones varies greatly, especially in the nasolabial region, due to a series of factors dependent upon each patient and the surgical technique used (Fig. 8.7). This variation makes it particularly difficult to find a soft-to-hard tissue ratio in the literature that applies to the cases we treat in daily practice. Therefore, the ideal way to achieve accuracy and provide a 3D planning that we consider "approximative" at best is by conducting studies in which the sample consists of patients undergoing surgical treatment by the same research team. This avoids biases regarding the surgical technique and patient characteristics.

Given that orthofacial planning is based on soft-tissue aesthetics, we have spent recent years reducing bias and avoiding the use of soft tissues in virtual planning. We have published a series of studies evaluating the effect of our minimally invasive surgical technique on controlling nasal enlargement and the definition of a soft-to-hard tissue ratio of this approach in surgical movements [8, 9].

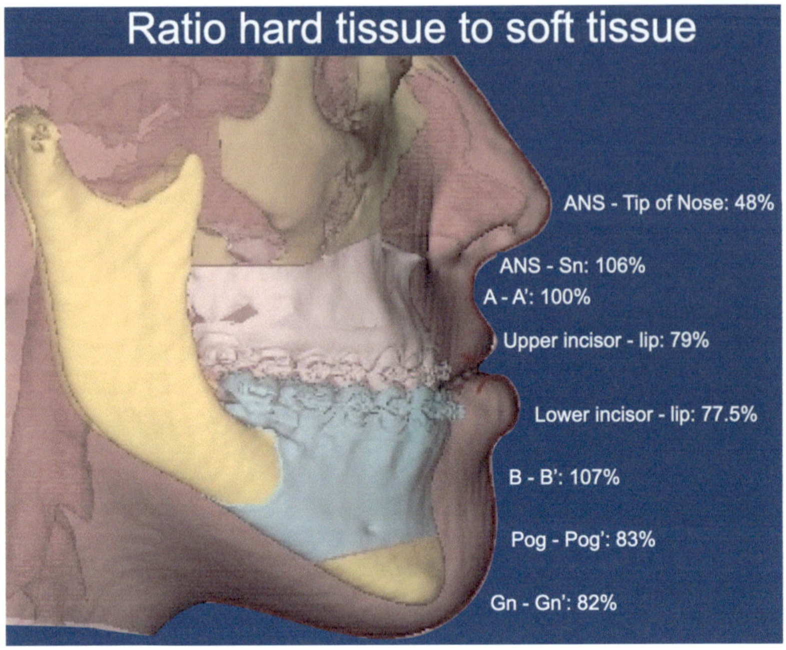

Fig. 8.8 Hard-to-soft tissue ratio: Nasolabial ratio and Mandible ratio

We found that patients undergoing segmented Le Fort I osteotomy had a 1.49 mm increase in interalar width, a 0.93 mm increase in alar base width, and a 1.54 mm increase in the upper lip length. Patients undergoing nonsegmented Le Fort I osteotomy had a 1.34 mm increase in interalar width, a 0.54 mm increase in alar base width, and a 1.41 mm increase in upper lip length [8]. Regarding the soft-tissue response to surgical movement, the pronasale followed the movement of the anterior nasal spine (ANS) in 48% of the cases, the subnasale followed the movement of the ANS in 106%, and the labrale superior followed the movement of the upper incisor in 79% of the cases [9] (Fig. 8.8).

In a mandibular soft-tissue prediction analysis, the number of variables affecting outcomes is significantly lower, resulting in a soft-to-hard tissue ratio of approximately 100% in the pogonion and of 78% between the lower lip and lower incisor. This makes 3D planning of this anatomical region much more predictable [10] (Fig. 8.8).

The information we collect from these studies is imported to the Dolphin 3D Imaging software (Dolphin Imaging & Management Solutions, Chatsworth, CA, USA), which we use for 3D planning—more specifically, into the "soft tissue rule editor" tool. Thus, we use the soft-to-hard tissue ratio obtained in our own studies when planning surgical movements (Fig. 8.9). In this way, we feel that we are getting closer to achieving optimal 3D planning in orthofacial surgery.

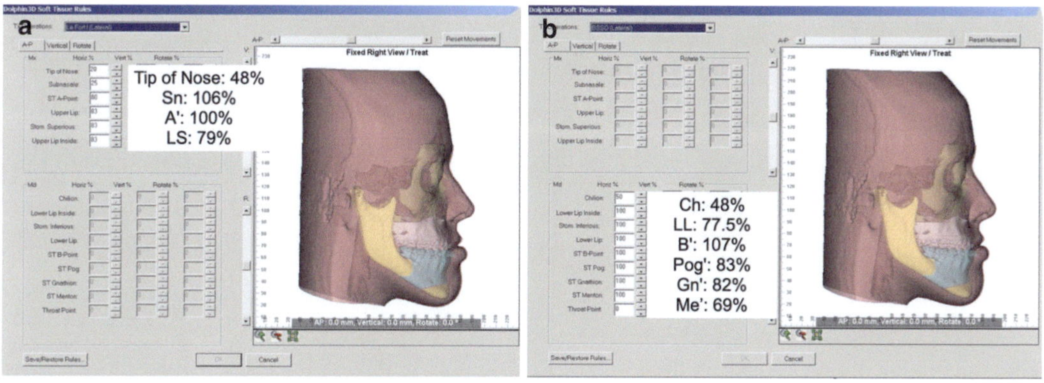

Fig. 8.9 Personalized soft-tissue rule. (**a**) Nasolabial; (**b**) Mandible

8.3 Three-Dimensional Planning and the Upper Airway

In a way similar to what occurs in soft-tissue 3D planning, the effect of orthognathic surgery upon the airway is not accurately predicted by software algorithms. However, the pharynx visualization and measurement tool plays an important role as a planning guide to increase the airway space and relieve obstruction in soft-tissue regions that may cause snoring and obstructive sleep apnea.

In relation to the diagnosis, the multiplanar sections of the upper airway (axial, coronal, and sagittal) are analyzed to assess the relationship between the dentofacial deformity and breathing difficulties of the patient. The nasopharynx, oropharynx, and hypopharynx are also examined in terms of volume and maximum constriction area [11] (Fig. 8.10). These data provide an extremely important reference regarding which type of surgery, whether bimaxillary advancement with a focus on the maxilla or mandible, is required.

All patients have their own individual needs, but through our research studies [12, 13], we obtained some important information that guides orthofacial surgery planning focusing on the upper airway. The mean airway dimension increase in maximum constriction areas with the maxillomandibular advancement surgery is 104%, which is far superior to that obtained with maxillary or mandibular advancement surgery alone. The volume increase is similar between monomaxillary and monomandibular advancement techniques: maxillary surgery increases the total volume by 26% and mostly benefits the nasopharynx and oropharynx, whereas mandibular surgery increases the total volume by 25% and mostly benefits the hypopharynx and oropharynx. Volume loss has been shown to occur 1 year after surgery and has been more associated with maxillomandibular and mandibular advancement techniques, meaning that the elastic effect of the suprahyoid muscles is directly related to the loss of benefits [12].

In an analysis of the surgical movements with the greatest impact upon the airway dimension increase, we ranked them in the following order of importance: (1) counterclockwise rotation of the maxillomandibular complex; (2) mandibular advancement; and (3) maxillary advancement. Chin advancement and downward movement of the posterior part of the maxilla are adjuvant surgical movements that enhance the effects of the three main ones. The downward movement of the entire maxilla and mandibular setback are the surgical movements with the greatest negative impact on the airway [12] (Fig. 8.11).

During surgical planning, we should always consider which surgical movements increase airflow capacity and decrease obstruction caused by the soft tissues of the soft palate, base of the tongue, and suprahyoid muscles. Therefore, a constriction area increase should be achieved to improve patient breathing, given that volume gain is a secondary goal, and only an intrapersonal parameter would identify whether orthofacial surgery has affected the airways.

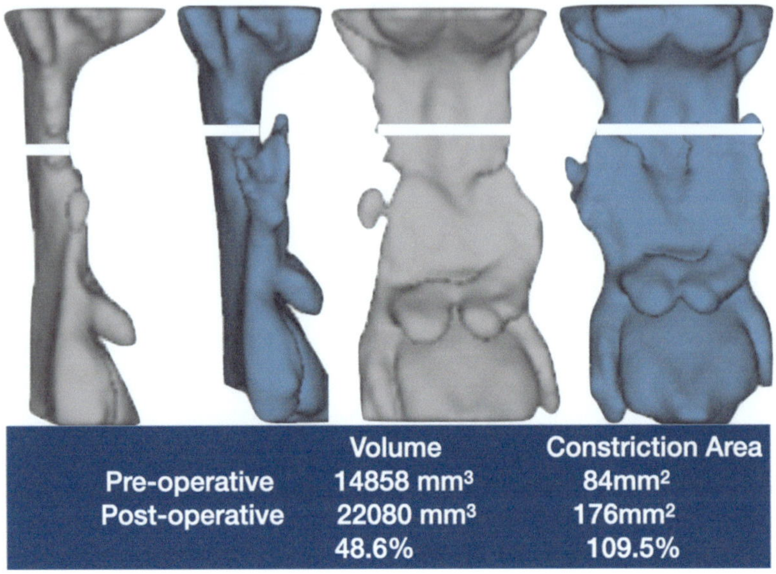

Fig. 8.10 Upper airway analysis. Gray—preoperative and blue—postoperative. White line—constriction area

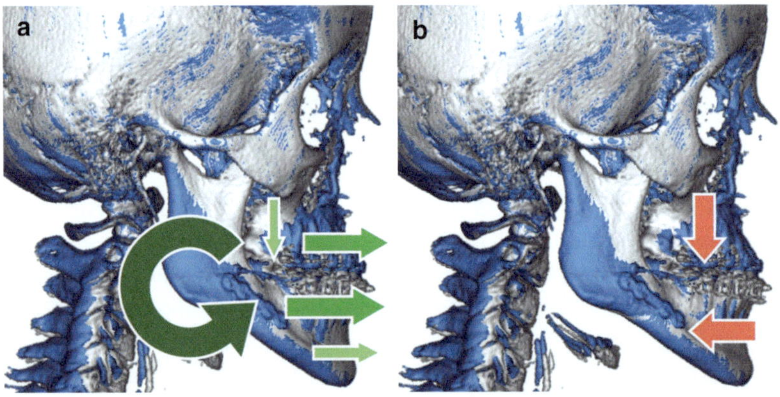

Fig. 8.11 Surgical movements' influence in the upper airway. (**a**) Most benefit; (**b**) Most damage

The airway of patients with respiratory complaints should be cleared as much as possible, especially in those with obstructive sleep apnea, but interference in patients without respiratory complaints should be kept to a minimum. This principle is also consistent with the aesthetic improvement provided by orthofacial surgery. Patients with maxillomandibular retrusion and facial flaccidity benefit from a reverse facelift caused by maxillomandibular advancement and counterclockwise rotation [14], and patients with mandibular prognathism and maxillary retrognathism benefit from maximum maxillary advancement and minimum or no mandibular setback.

8.4 Auxiliary 3D Tools for Orthofacial Surgery

Some 3D tools are essential for constant improvement of surgical techniques and aesthetic/functional outcomes. To this end, we believe that protocols for imaging superimposition should be used to evaluate surgical outcomes; personalized cutting guides improve the results in complex situations, and 3D photographs are a good tool for planning orthofacial surgery together with the patient.

8.4.1 Superimposition of 3D Imaging

Superimposition of 3D imaging is a fundamental tool in the evolution of orthofacial surgery, as it provides feedback after each procedure and promotes surgical self-knowledge. It is also the basis of all of our clinical studies, in which we evaluate surgical outcomes in terms of facial aesthetics, respiratory function, and planning accuracy. Thus, this tool has certainly added more predictability to our procedures.

As a rule, we use a protocol created for imaging superimposition with the Dolphin 3D Imaging software (Dolphin Imaging & Management Solutions, Chatsworth, CA, USA)—the same software we use for virtual planning. The protocol is based on CBCT scan voxels, and the overlay is performed on the anterior base of the skull, given that this structure is not affected by orthognathic surgery. Postoperative and preoperative CBCT scans are superimposed for an analysis of the impact of orthofacial surgery (Fig. 8.12).

The total superimposition time is approximately 3 min and 20 s. The protocol is fully reproducible and has an accuracy of 0.2 mm, meaning that it is a user-friendly tool that could be used routinely in private practice [15, 16].

8.4.2 Cutting Guides

We believe that the correction of facial asymmetries represents the most complex treatment in orthofacial surgery. Thus, we use cutting guides that make the osteotomy more precise and the treatment more objective.

We can treat complex cases such as condylar hyperplasia with intraoral proportional condylectomy combined with orthognathic surgery thanks to a cutting guide that we developed to achieve bilateral symmetry in the dimensions of the mandibular rami. These guides ensure that all active or pathological parts of the mandibular condyle are removed and that the mandibular angles will be at the same height after the surgical procedure. Therefore, surgical treatment can now be performed in a single step, which was not possible via an intraoral access [17] (Fig. 8.13).

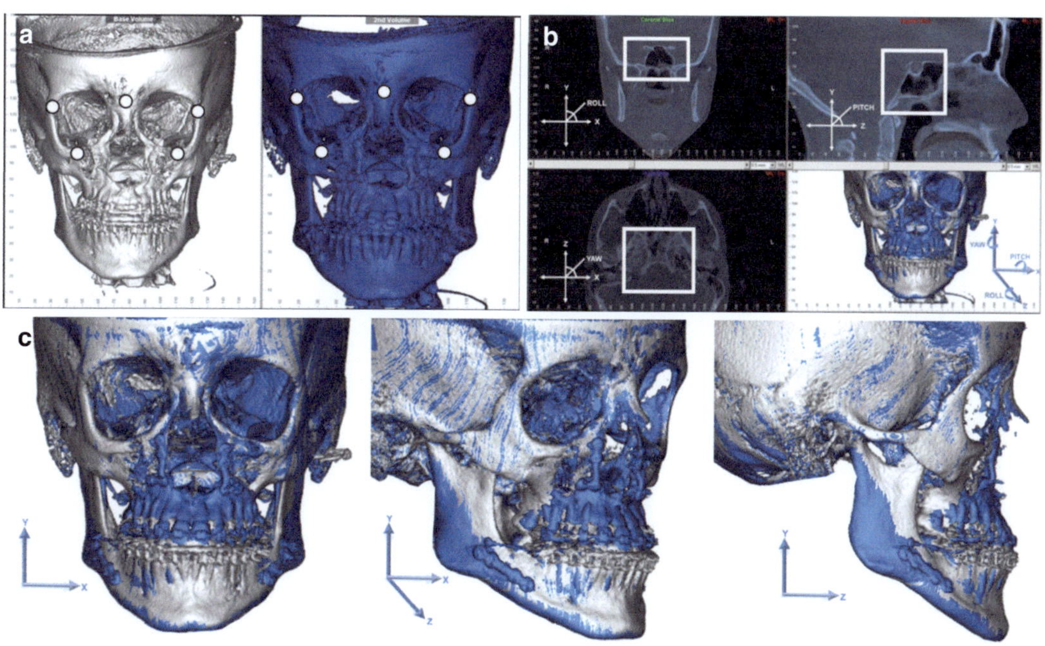

Fig. 8.12 Pre- and post-superimposition. (**a**) First step, landmark superimposition; (**b**) Second step, voxel-based superimposition; (**c**) Superimposition result

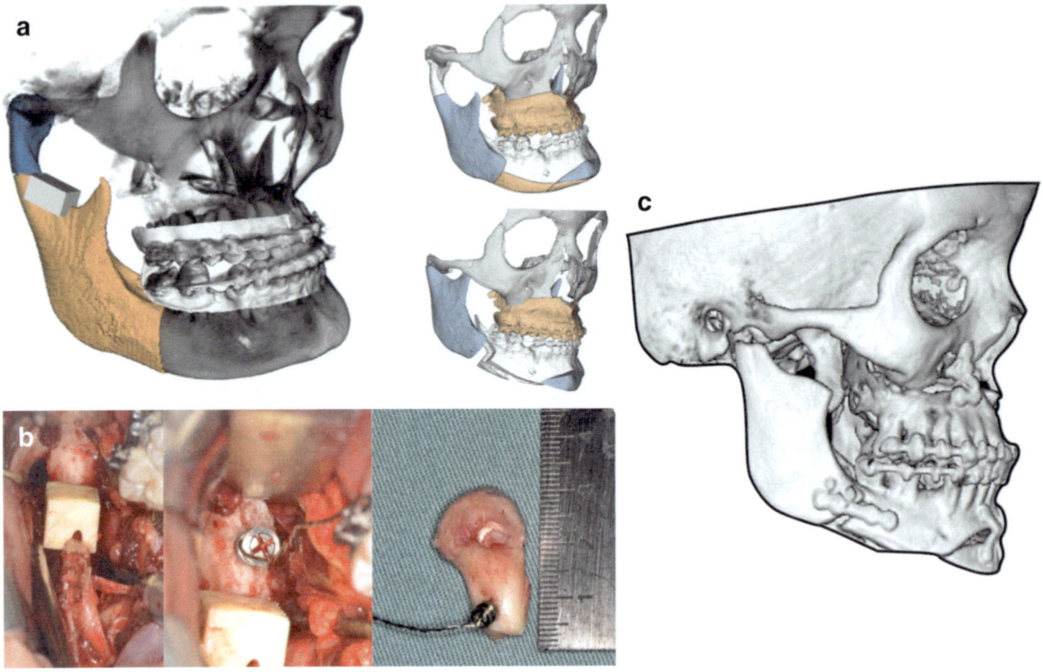

Fig. 8.13 Intraoral proportional condylectomy. (**a**) 3D planning; (**b**) Surgical technique; (**c**) Postoperative 3D imaging

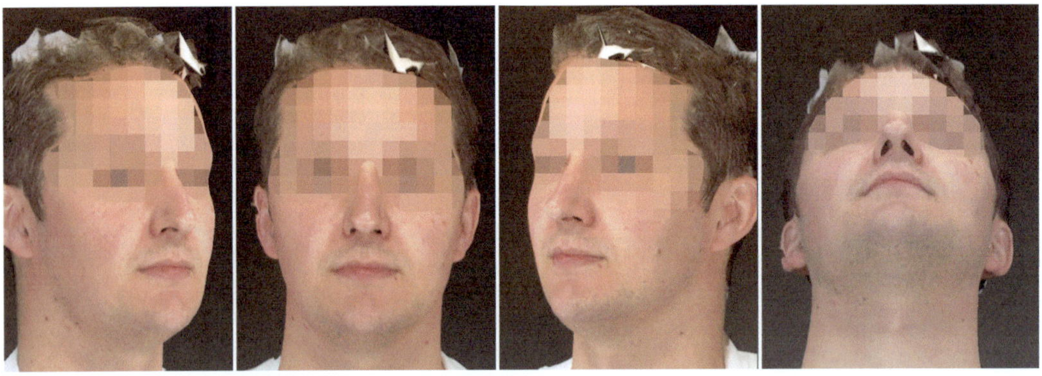

Fig. 8.14 Facial 3D imaging

8.4.3 Three-Dimensional Photographs

Three-dimensional photography is an excellent tool for diagnosis, planning, and postoperative control in orthofacial surgery. It is used to evaluate facial soft tissue and to convey more reality to the virtual model generated by virtual planning, which makes it easier for patients to visualize the procedure and recognize their faces.

Thus, 3D imaging of the soft tissues can be used as a research tool to evaluate the aesthetic outcomes of the procedure and as an auxiliary tool to facial analysis in clinical practice [18] (Fig. 8.14).

References

1. Hernández-Alfaro F, Giralt-Hernando M, Brabyn PJ, Haas OL Jr, Valls-Ontañón A. Variation between natural head orientation and Frankfort horizontal planes in orthognathic surgery patients: 187 consecutive cases. Int J Oral Maxillofac Surg. 2021;50(9):1226–32.
2. Hernández-Alfaro F. Upper incisor to Soft Tissue Plane (UI-STP). A new reference for diagnosis and planning in dentofacial deformities. Med Oral Patol Oral Cir Bucal. 2010;15(5):e779–81.
3. Hernández-Alfaro F, Guijarro-Martínez R. New protocol for three-dimensional surgical planning and CAD/CAM splint generation in orthognathic surgery: an in vitro and in vivo study. Int J Oral Maxillofac Surg. 2013;42(12):1547–56.
4. Aboul-Hosn Centenero S, Hernández-Alfaro F. 3D planning in orthognathic surgery: CAD/CAM surgical splints and prediction of the soft and hard tissues results: our experience in 16 cases. J Craniofac Surg. 2012;40(2):162–8.
5. Haas OL Jr, Becker OE, de Oliveira RB. Computer-aided planning in orthognathic surgery—systematic review. Int J Oral Maxillofac Surg. 2015;44:329–42.
6. de Sousa P, Gil A, Guijarro-Martínez V, Haas OL Jr, Hernández-Alfaro F. Three-dimensional analysis of nasolabial soft tissue changes after Le Fort I osteotomy: a systematic review of the literature. Int J Oral Maxillofac Surg. 2019;48(9):1185–200.
7. Hertanto M, Ayoub AF, Benington PCM, Naudi KB, McKenzie PS. Orthognathic patient perception of 3D facial soft tissue prediction planning. J Craniomaxillofac Surg. 2021;49(9):783–8.
8. de Sousa P, Gil A, Guijarro-Martínez R, Haas OL Jr, Masià-Gridilla J, Valls-Ontañón A, Belle de Oliveira R, Hernández-Alfaro F. Nasolabial soft tissue effects of segmented and non-segmented Le Fort I osteotomy using a modified alar cinch technique-a cone beam computed tomography evaluation. Int J Oral Maxillofac Surg. 2020;49(7):889–94.
9. de Sousa P, Gil A, Machado-Fernández A, Guijarro-Martínez R, Hernández-Alfaro F, Haas OL Jr, Belle de Oliveira R. Le Fort I osteotomy and soft tissue response: a retrospective cohort study comparing three different techniques. J Craniofac Surg. 2022;50(2):107–13.
10. Lisboa CO, Martins MM, Ruellas ACO, Ferreira DMTP, Maia LC, MattosTC. Soft tissue assessment before and after mandibular advancement or setback surgery using three-dimensional images: systematic review and meta-analysis. Int J Oral Maxillofac Surg. 2018;47(11):1389–97.
11. Guijarro-Martínez R, Swennen GRJ. Three-dimensional cone beam computed tomography definition of the anatomical subregions of the upper airway: a validation study. Int J Oral Maxillofac Surg. 2013;42:1140.
12. Giralt-Hernando M, Valls-Ontañón A, Haas OL Jr, Masià-Gridilla J, Hernández-Alfaro F. What are the surgical movements in orthognathic surgery that most affect the upper airways? A three-dimensional analysis. J Oral Maxillofac Surg. 2021;79(2):450–62.
13. Giralt-Hernando M, Valls-Ontañón A, Guijarro-Martínez R, Masià-Gridilla J, Hernández-Alfaro F. Impact of surgical maxillomandibular advancement upon pharyngeal airway volume and the apnoea-hypopnoea index in the treatment of obstructive sleep apnoea: systematic review and meta-analysis. BMJ Open Resp Res. 2019;9;6(1):e000402.
14. Lorente C, Hernández-Alfaro F, Perez-Vela M, Lorente P, Lorente T. Surgical-orthodontic approach for facial rejuvenation based on a reverse facelift. Prog Orthod. 2019;26;20(1):34.
15. Haas OL Jr, Guijarro-Martínez R, de Sousa P, Gil A, Méndez-Manjón I, Valls-Ontañón A, Belle de Oliveira R, Hernández-Alfaro F. Cranial base superimposition of cone-beam computed tomography images. J Craniofac Surg. 2019;30(6):1809–14.
16. Andriola FO, Haas OL Jr, Guijarro-Martínez R, Hernández-Alfaro F, de Oliveira RB, Pagnoncelli RM, Swennen GRJ. Computed tomography imaging superimposition protocols to assess outcomes in orthognathic surgery: a systematic review with comprehensive recommendations. Dentomaxillofac Radiol. 2022;1;51(3):20210340.
17. Haas OL Jr, Fariña RS, Hernández-Alfaro F, de Oliveira RB. Minimally invasive intraoral proportional condylectomy with a three-dimensionally printed cutting guide. Int J Oral Maxillofac Surg. 2020;49(11):1435–8.
18. Wampfler JJ, Gkantidis N. Superimposition of serial 3-dimensional facial photographs to assess changes over time: a systematic review. Am J Orthod Dentofacial Orthop. 2022;161:182–97.

Minimally Invasive Surgery of the Maxilla

9

Federico Hernández-Alfaro

9.1 Introduction

The classical and most frequent maxillary osteotomy is the Le Fort I technique [1, 2]. Years ago, we designed and published a minimally invasive Le Fort I osteotomy allowing mobilization of the maxilla, adopting a reduced approach and a special maneuver to provoke pterygomaxillary disjunction [3]. Later, we designed an ancillary procedure to facilitate the technique through a transmucosal pterygomaxillary osteotomy using a piezoelectric saw [3].

In our experience, this technique [3] has proved useful for any type of clinical scenario, irrespective of the direction and amount of maxillary repositioning.

9.2 Technique

After infiltration with saline solution plus lidocaine and epinephrine, we need a caliper to take the only measurement needed during the entire bimaxillary procedure, namely the vertical distance between the internal canthus and the orthodontic arch (or a mini-screw in the event of a case managed with aligners or lingual orthodontics) (Fig. 9.1).

The amount of vertical repositioning of the bimaxillary complex indeed is the only information not contained in the splints, and in fact, it is only of relative value, since the ultimate fine-tuning of vertical maxillary repositioning is decided during surgery itself, analyzing the reaction of the upper lip to maxillary advancement and/or rotations [4]. Again, this is one of the reasons why I do not like customized plates, which do not allow for these intraoperative decisions.

Our first move in maxillary surgery is to perform transmucosal pterygomaxillary disjunction with a piezoelectric device [5]. This very simple and straightforward maneuver [4, 5] has proved very effective combined with our previously published "twist technique" [3] in achieving clean downfracturing of the maxilla. We initially designed and published a three-dimensional (3D) guiding system to perform this posterior osteotomy [6]. Later, after completing the learning curve, we found the use of this guide to be unnecessary. Instead, on the cone-beam computed tomography (CBCT) scan, we measure the distance between the pterygoid hamulus and the pterygomaxillary disjunction and use this reference intraoperatively to find the appropriate place for the insertion of the piezoelectric inset (Fig. 9.2a and b).

Through a minimally invasive incision from lateral incisor to lateral incisor, we cut the anterior

F. Hernández-Alfaro (✉)
Department of Oral and Maxillofacial Surgery, International University of Catalonia, Barcelona, Spain
e-mail: h.alfaro@uic.es

F. Hernández-Alfaro, A. Valls Ontañón (eds.), *Orthofacial Surgery*,
https://doi.org/10.1007/978-3-031-76185-0_9

border of the nasal muscles. Periosteal elevation of the anterior and lateral walls of the maxilla to the pterygoid region is then performed to this small incision [7] (Fig. 9.3).

The nasal spine is osteotomized from the maxilla with the piezoelectric saw. After this subspinal osteotomy, the nasal mucosa is detached from the nasal floor with a periosteal elevator. Using the latter, the nasal septum is luxated laterally to separate it from the nasal crest of the maxilla (Fig. 9.4).

If segmental osteotomies of the maxilla are planned, we like to perform the interdental parts at this point. These are performed with the piezoelectric saw in a descending fashion with minimal periosteal elevation. In any case, to avoid periodontal problems, it is important to preserve the periosteum under the keratinized mucosa attached to the bone (Fig. 9.5).

Subsequently, standard Le Fort I horizontal osteotomies are performed using a reciprocating saw with a 4 cm blade. Posteriorly, the cut is slanted slightly downward toward the maxillary tuberosity. The medial walls of the maxillary sinuses are cut as the reciprocating saw proceeds medially. Lateral osteotomies are completed by driving a sharp, straight 2 cm osteotome from the nasal crest of the maxilla to the pterygomaxillary junction (Fig. 9.6).

Classical pterygomaxillary disjunction from a lateral approach (i.e., driving a curved osteotome at the pterygomaxillary fissure) is not performed. Instead, a straight wedged (1.5 cm wide) osteotome is driven through the horizontal osteotomy from the pyriform buttress back to the junction (Fig. 9.7a and b).

Unlike classical pterygomaxillary disjunction, which entails a lateral approach to the pterygomaxillary fissure with a curved osteotome, the twist technique [3] seeks to achieve pterygomaxillary disjunction from a frontal approach with a straight osteotome.

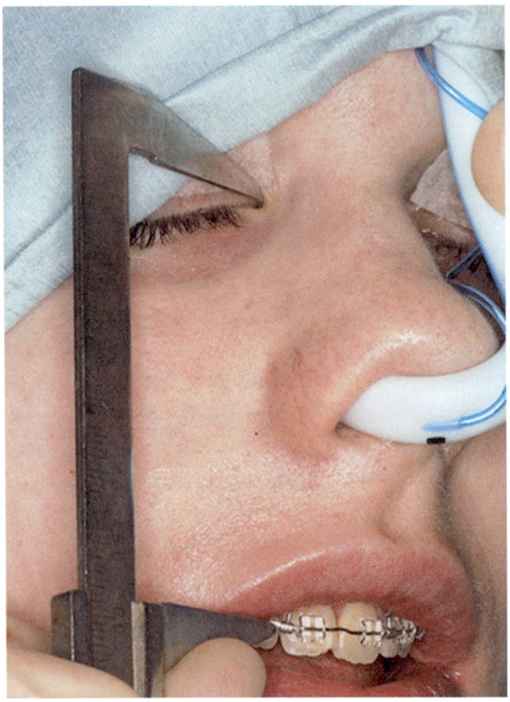

Fig. 9.1 Distance between the orthodontic arch and internal canthus is the only measurement needed in bimaxillary surgery. The rest of the information is contained in the splints. Measurement of the arch–internal canthus distance

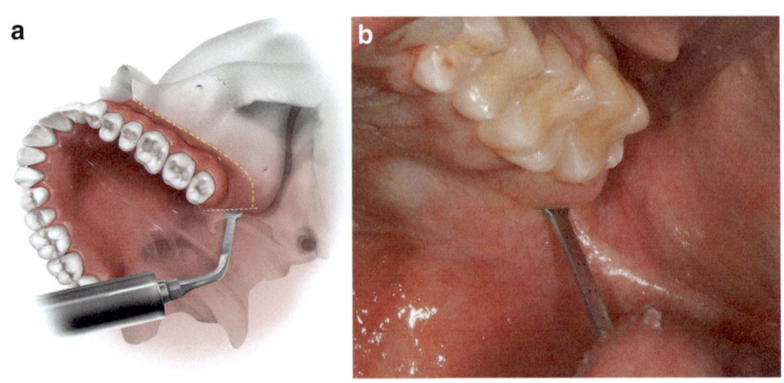

Fig. 9.2 (**a** and **b**) We start our Le Fort I osteotomy by performing transmucosal disjunction of the pterygomaxillary junction with a piezoelectric device

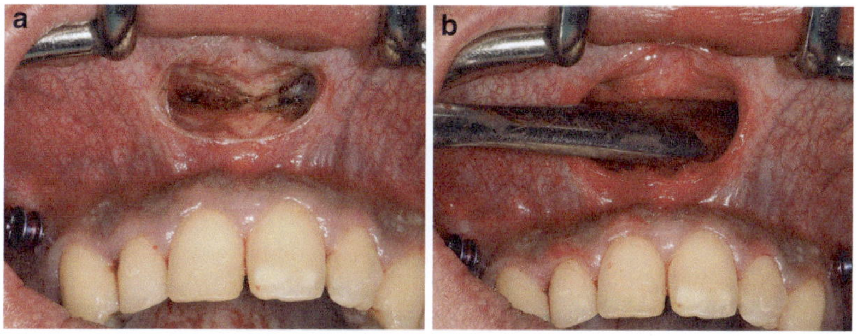

Fig. 9.3 (**a** and **b**) Through a minimally invasive incision from lateral incisor to lateral incisor, the anterior border of the nasal muscles is cut. Periosteal elevation of the anterior and lateral walls of the maxilla to the pterygoid region is performed to this small incision

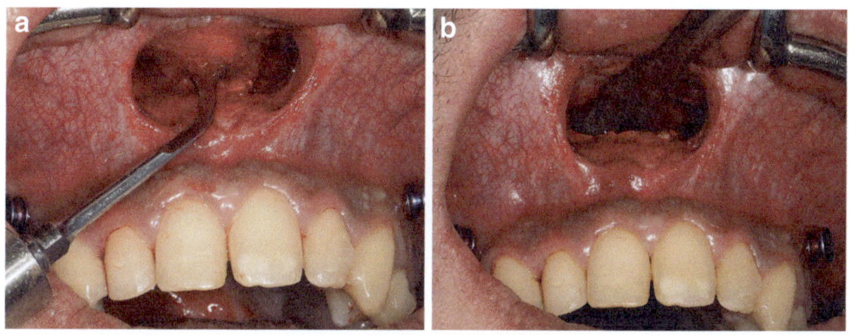

Fig. 9.4 (**a**) Subspinal osteotomy. (**b**) Elevation of the nasal mucosa

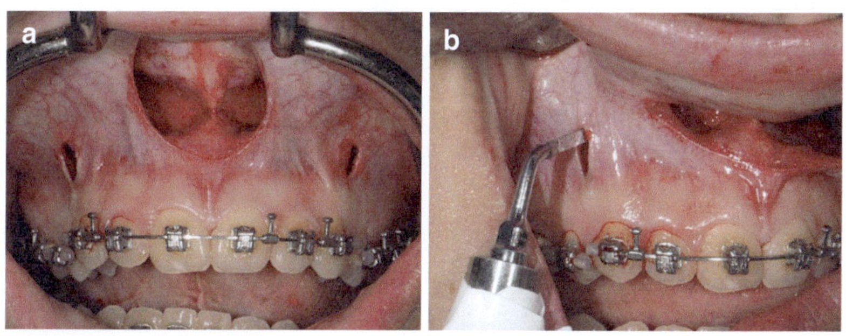

Fig. 9.5 (**a** and **b**) If interdental segmentation is performed between cuspid and bicuspid, we add two small stab incisions instead of prolonging the main access

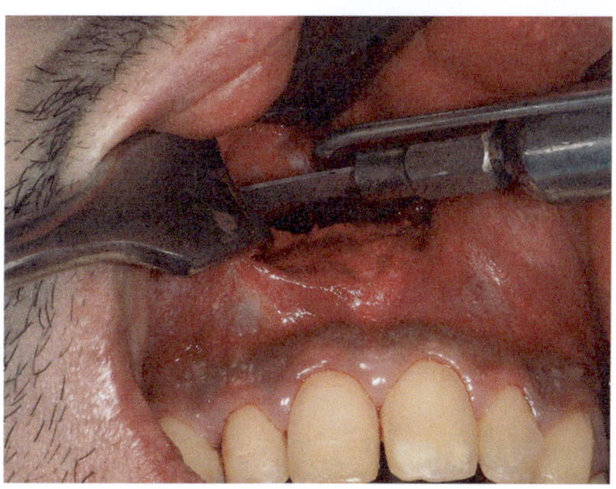

Fig. 9.6 Horizontal osteotomy is performed with a reciprocating saw

Downfracture is achieved by inwardly rotating the osteotome that has been previously fixed at the zygomatic buttress, sliding the osteotome backward along the lateral osteotomies (Fig. 9.8).

Separation of the maxilla is completed instantly. Successful maxillary separation from the cranial base can be verified under excellent direct vision, and the greater palatine neurovascular bundle can be easily dissected. Lateral vision is adequate to enable balanced elimination of bony interferences and ensure good bone-to-bone contact.

This modified approach allows a substantially smaller soft-tissue incision (2.8 cm on average)

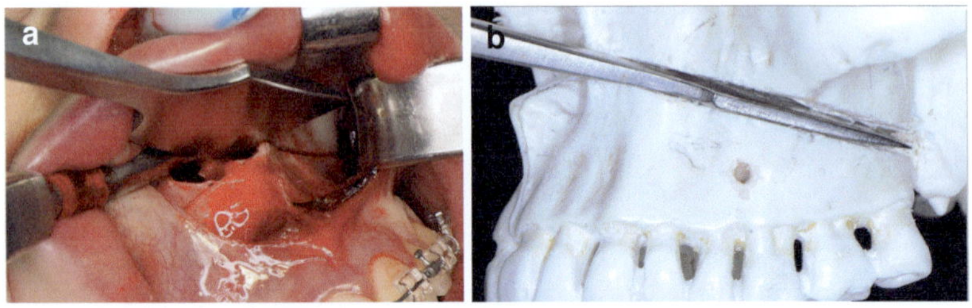

Fig. 9.7 (**a** and **b**) Our "twist technique" is initiated by sliding a 2 cm wide osteotome along the horizontal osteotomy

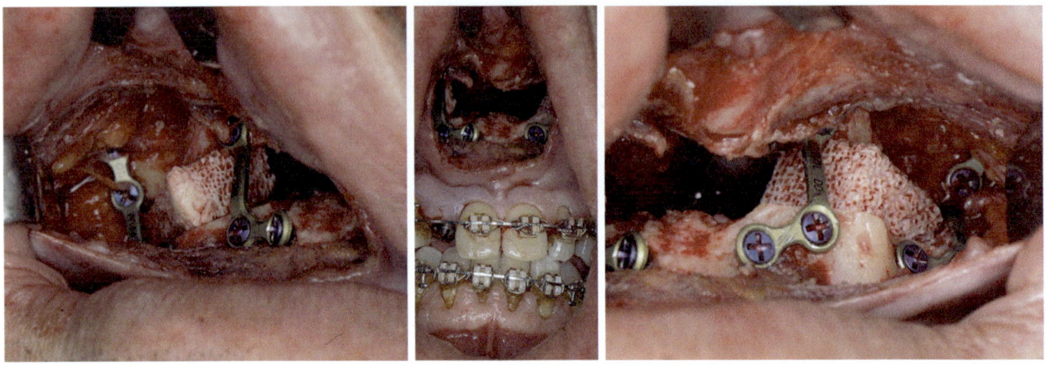

Fig. 9.8 Once the pterygomaxillary region is reached, an internal twist provokes downfracturing of the maxilla

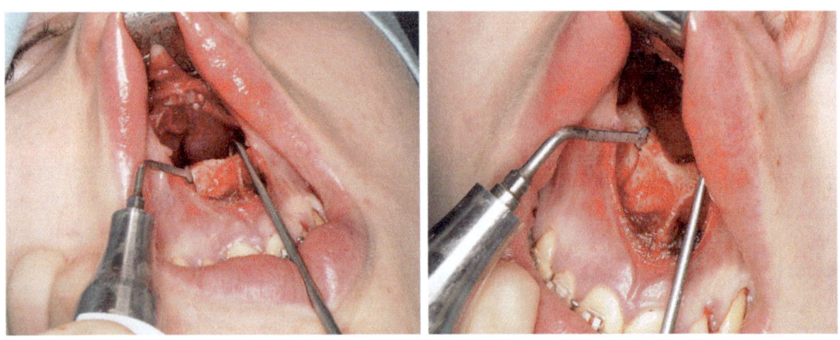

Fig. 9.9 Segmentation of the premaxilla

than the classical "molar-to-molar" exposure. The risk of ischemic events is minimized by the preservation of most of the vascular supply to the bone through the buccal corridors (Fig. 9.9). In addition, the final visible scar on the buccal mucosa is significantly smaller. It must be noted, however, that decreasing the incision length should be considered a technical progression from the classical approach and not a primary goal for the inexperienced orthognathic surgeon. That said, the twist technique is technically undemanding and is taught at our center as a standard method for pterygomaxillary disjunction.

Potential severe complications after pterygomaxillary disjunction have been reported in the scientific literature [8–12]. Many of these complications have been caused by malpositioning the osteotome or by accidental fractures during maxillary downfracture [9]. Although several technical modifications have been proposed to minimize the risk of pterygoid process fracture [12–20], studies of strain distribution with different osteotome designs have indicated that pterygoid plate fractures are likely to occur regardless of the type of osteotome used [21]. Similarly, fractures occur, irrespective of whether a pterygoid chisel is used or not [12]. In any case, a pterygoid plate fracture should not be considered a complication because it is not necessarily the cause of hemorrhage or nerve injury [12].

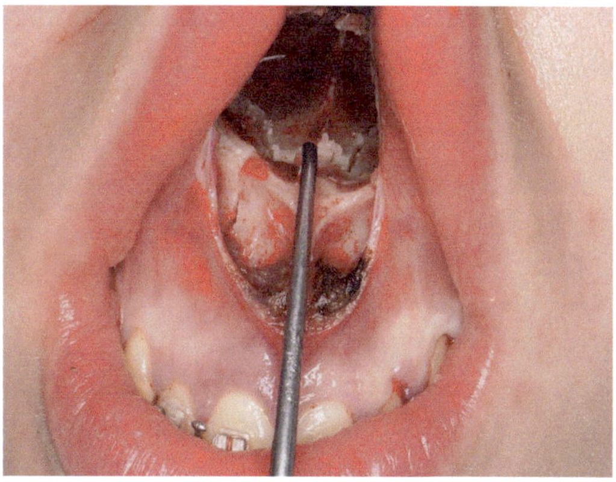

Fig. 9.10 Completion of segmentation and full mobilization of segments

Once the maxilla is downfractured and mobilized, if segmentation needs to be made, interdental osteotomies are continued posteriorly with the piezoelectric saw and with two paramedial cuts in the floor of the mouth. They are then connected with an additional horizontal cut behind the nasomaxillary foramen, thus producing a four-piece maxilla (Fig. 9.10).

After 3D repositioning the maxilla into occlusion with the mandible through the final splint, vertical adjustment is made using the caliper and modifying the original distance according to the desired vertical movement.

Maxillary fixation is usually achieved with two preformed miniplates (Fig. 9.11) [22]. Only in cases of segmentation with large expansion might we use four standard plates, always leaving the anterior maxillary segment free [23] to allow for postsurgical orthodontic management (i.e., torque change and/or maximizing overbite) (Fig. 9.12).

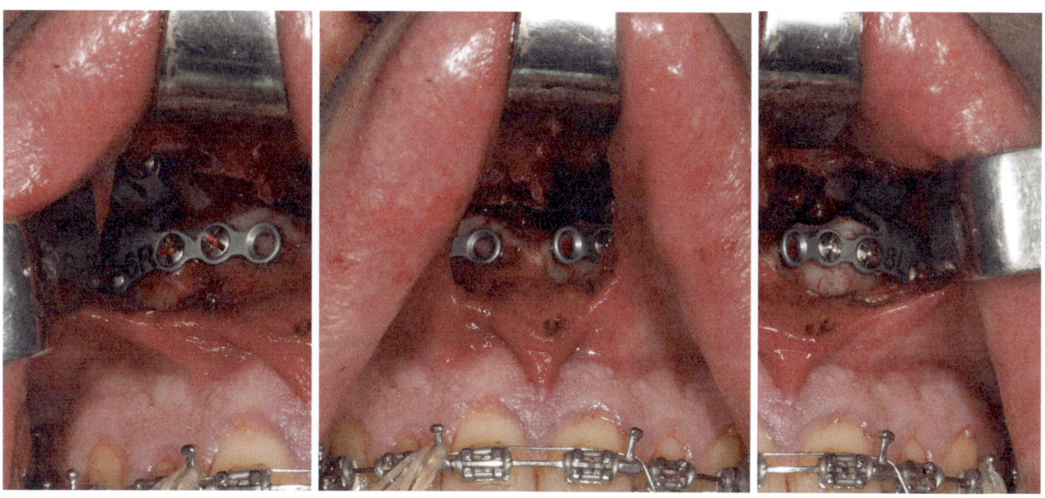

Fig. 9.11 Once the maxillary segments are repositioned into the final splint, maxillary fixation takes place

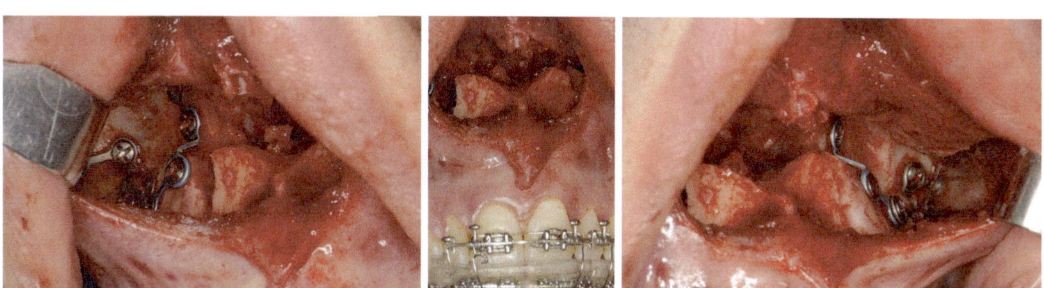

Fig. 9.12 If large expansions are performed, four miniplates are used

Grafting should be applied in all significant (>3 mm) gaps. Our material of choice is hydroxyapatite in blocks, which can be easily trimmed and adapted wherever necessary [24].

These blocks are especially important in maxillary downgrafting and/or counterclockwise rotational movements of the maxilla and also as fillers in segmentation spaces, typically between laterals and canines (Fig. 9.13).

Suturing is as important as the access. With our minimally invasive incision, we aim at preserving most of the paranasal muscles, and ideally only the myrtiformis muscles should be cut. When closing, the four stumps of the muscles are sutured in cross-fashion with 4/0 Vicryl [25] (Figs. 9.14 and 9.15).

This published technique allows maximum preservation of nasal width, as also evidenced by the results of our clinical studies [7].

Finally, the mucosa is sutured in V/Y fashion with 5/0 Vicryl.

It must be noted that, when indicated, third molar extraction is always performed from an occlusal approach before the Le Fort I procedure, though it is our preference to have all wisdom teeth removed at least 6 months before surgery.

The twist technique [3] of pterygomaxillary disjunction, combined with transmucosal pterygomaxillary disjunction, is a safe and efficient technical modification for maxillary downfracture [3, 5]. In our experience, no particular limitations or contraindications apply with this technique.

Compared with classical pterygomaxillary disjunction, the twist technique uses a frontal approach and a straight osteotome. Downfracture is achieved by inwardly rotating the osteotome that has been fixed at the zygomatic buttress. This modified approach allows a substantially smaller soft-tissue incision, achieves immediate effective separation of the maxilla, and affords adequate

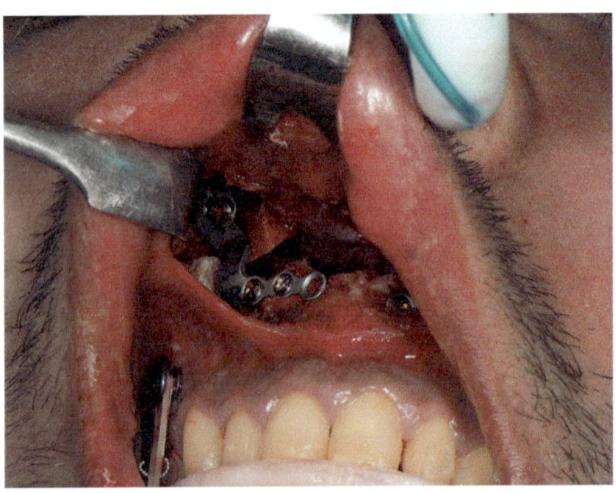

Fig. 9.13 One-piece maxilla with downgrafting. See the anterior portion of the hydroxyapatite block

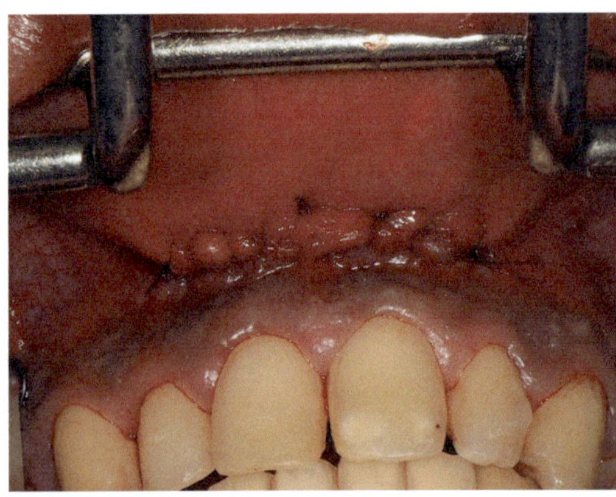

Fig. 9.15 The mucosa is sutured with a 5/0 reabsorbable monofilament

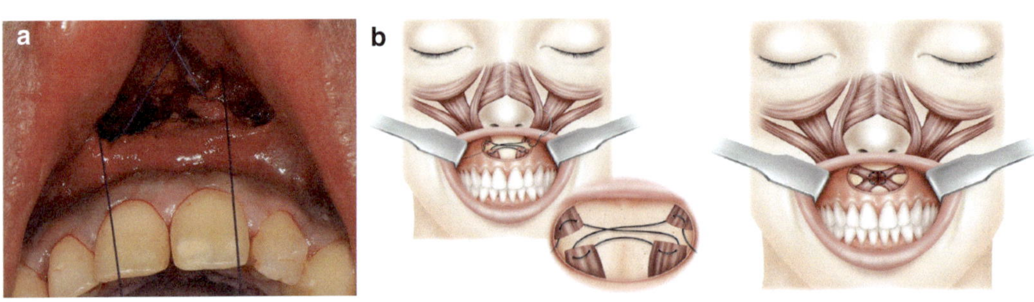

Fig. 9.14 (**a** and **b**). Cross-suturing of the nasal muscles with 4/0 Vicryl

visualization of the greater palatine neurovascular bundle. Preliminary experience in over 2500 patients indicates that the procedure meets the necessary requirements of safety and technical accuracy [3, 5].

9.3 Patient-Specific Implants and Minimally Invasive Le Fort I

Personalized medicine and surgery has emerged in different fields of medicine and dentistry. Patient-specific cutting guides and plates have been advocated in the last few years as a means to improve accuracy and reduce surgical times in orthognathic surgery. The drawback of this new technology, however, is that it requires oversized hardware which is incompatible with our minimally invasive surgical approaches.

Two years ago, we started a new project with a clear goal in mind: to develop miniaturized patient-specific hardware which could be applied maintaining our reduced approaches to Le Fort I osteotomy.

With this aim, we developed a novel design of small puzzle-connected cutting guides which perfectly and easily adapt to the anterior nasal spine and piriform aperture on each side (Fig. 9.16).

Fully customized plates at the piriform buttress are used to fix the maxilla after completing our minimally invasive Le Fort I osteotomy. These plates contain all the information on the 3D repositioning of the maxilla and are fixed with screws which (thanks to the custom design from the computed tomography scan) engage in the thicker areas of the buttress (Fig. 9.17).

We performed and published a proof-of-concept study in five consecutive patients managed with our novel design of cutting guides and plates. The study revealed accuracy figures similar to those published in the literature using the classical oversized hardware [26].

We have been using this new system for a year now, and we feel there is no turning back, since it successfully combines our minimally invasive surgical principles with full customization.

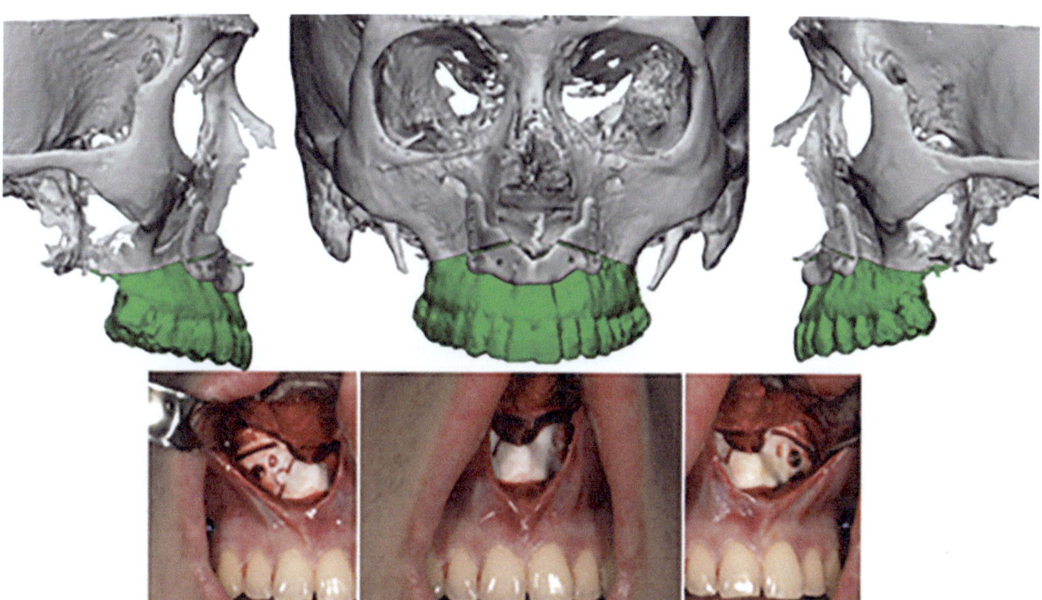

Fig. 9.16 Miniaturized puzzle-connected cutting guides

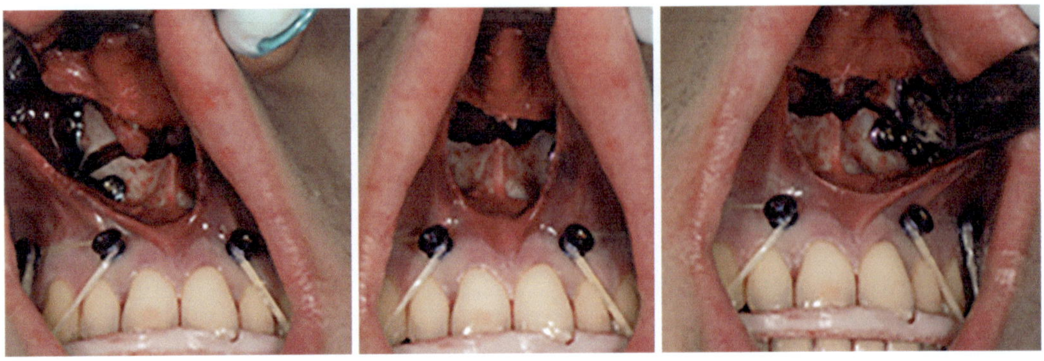

Fig. 9.17 Fully customized rigid plates applied at the piriform buttress

References

1. Bell WH. Le Forte I osteotomy for correction of maxillary deformities. J Oral Surg. 1975;33(6):412–26.
2. Epker BN. Vascular considerations in orthognathic surgery. II. Maxillary osteotomies. Oral Surg Oral Med Oral Pathol. 1984;57(5):473–8.
3. Hernandez-Alfaro F, Guijarro-Martinez R. "Twist technique" for pterygomaxillary dysjunction in minimally invasive Le Fort I osteotomy. J Oral Maxillofac Surg. 2013;71(2):389–92.
4. Valls-Ontañón A, Hernández-Margarit P, Mazarro-Campos A, Hernández-Alfaro F. Transmucosal posterior segmentation in the context of minimally invasive Le Fort I osteotomy: technical note. J Stomatol Oral Maxillofac Surg France. 2022;123:e82–4.
5. Hernández-Alfaro F, Ghuloom M, Giralt-Hernando M, Lázaro-Abdulkarim A, Valls-Ontañón A. Transmucosal pterygomaxillary disjunction using a piezoelectric device, in the context of the minimally invasive Le Fort I osteotomy protocol. Int J Oral Maxillofac Surg. 2022;52:569.
6. Hernández Alfaro F, Paternostro Betancourt D, Haas Junior OL, Valls Ontañón A. Customized guide for transmucosal pterygomaxillary disjunction: proof of concept. J Stomatol Oral Maxillofac Surg. 2022;000:3–6.
7. de Sousa Gil AP, Guijarro-Martínez R, Haas OLJ, Masià-Gridilla J, Valls-Ontañón A, de Oliveira RB, et al. Nasolabial soft tissue effects of segmented and non-segmented Le Fort I osteotomy using a modified alar cinch technique-a cone beam computed tomography evaluation. Int J Oral Maxillofac Surg. 2020;49(7):889–94.
8. Lanigan DT, Hey JH, West RA. Major vascular complications of orthognathic surgery: hemorrhage associated with Le Fort I osteotomies. J Oral Maxillofac Surg. 1990;48(6):561–73.
9. Ueki K, Nakagawa K, Marukawa K, Yamamoto E. Le Fort I osteotomy using an ultrasonic bone curette to fracture the pterygoid plates. J Craniomaxillofac Surg. 2004;32(6):381–6.
10. Precious DS, Morrison A, Ricard D. Pterygomaxillary separation without the use of an osteotome. J Oral Maxillofac Surg. 1991;49(1):98–9.
11. Robinson PP, Hendy CW. Pterygoid plate fractures caused by the Le Fort I osteotomy. Br J Oral Maxillofac Surg. 1986;24(3):198–202.
12. Precious DS, Goodday RH, Bourget L, Skulsky FG. Pterygoid plate fracture in Le Fort I osteotomy with and without pterygoid chisel: a computed tomography scan evaluation of 58 patients. J Oral Maxillofac Surg. 1993;51(2):151–3.
13. Dupont C, Ciaburro TH, Prévost Y. Simplifying the Le Fort I type of maxillary osteotomy. Plast Reconstr Surg. 1974;54(2):142–7.
14. Trimble LD, Tideman H, Stoelinga PJ. A modification of the pterygoid plate separation in low-level maxillary osteotomies. J Oral Maxillofac Surg. 1983;41(8):544–6.
15. Wikkeling OM, Tacoma J. Osteotomy of the pterygomaxillary junction. Int J Oral Surg. 1975;4(3):99–103.
16. Cheng LH, Robinson PP. Evaluation of a swan's neck osteotome for pterygomaxillary dysjunction in the Le Fort I osteotomy. Br J Oral Maxillofac Surg. 1993;31(1):52–3.
17. Thieme G, Stuttgart V, York N. Pterygoid plate separation using an oscillating saw in Le Fort I osteotomy technical note. J Craniomaxillofac Surg. 1991;19:153–4.
18. Laster Z, Ardekian L, Rachmiel A, Peled M. Use of the "shark-fin" osteotome in separation of the pterygomaxillary junction in Le Fort I osteotomy: a clinical and computerized tomography study. Int J Oral Maxillofac Surg. 2002;31(1):100–3.
19. Stajcić Z. Altering the angulation of a curved osteotome--does it have effects on the type of pterygomaxillary disjunction in Le Fort I osteotomy? An experimental study. Int J Oral Maxillofac Surg. 1991;20(5):301–3.
20. Lanigan DT, Loewy J. Postoperative computed tomography scan study of the pterygomaxillary separation during the Le Fort I osteotomy using a micro-oscillating saw. J Oral Maxillofac Surg. 1995;53(10):1161–6.

21. Hiranuma Y, Yamamoto Y, Iizuka T. Strain distribution during separation of the pterygomaxillary suture by osteotomes. Comparison between Obwegeser's osteotome and swan's neck osteotome. J Craniomaxillofac Surg. 1988;16(1):13–7.
22. Susarla SM, Ettinger R, Preston K, Kapadia H, Egbert MA. Two-point nasomaxillary fixation of the Le Fort I osteotomy: assessment of stability at one year postoperative. Int J Oral Maxillofac Surg. 2020 Apr;49(4):466–70.
23. Haas Junior OL, Guijarro-Martínez R, de Sousa Gil AP, da Silva ML, de Oliveira RB, Hernández-Alfaro F. Stability and surgical complications in segmental Le Fort I osteotomy: a systematic review [internet]. Int J Oral Maxillofac Surg Elsevier. 2017;46:1071–87. [cited 2017 Jul 2]. Available from: http://www.ncbi.nlm.nih.gov/pubmed/28601432
24. Haas Junior OL, da Silva ML, Scolari N, Emmel Becker O, Fernandes Santos Melo M, Belle de Oliveira R. Bone grafting with granular biomaterial in segmental maxillary osteotomy: a case report. Int J Surg Case Rep. 2016;25(June):238–42.
25. Hernández-Alfaro F, Paredes de Sousa Gil A, Haas Junior OL, Masià-Gridilla J, Valls-Ontañón A, Guijarro-Martinez R. [Soft tissue management to control nasal changes after Le Fort I osteotomy]. Orthod Fr. 2017;88(4):343–6.
26. Hernández-Alfaro F, Saavedra O, Duran-Valles F, Valls-Ontañón A. On the feasibility of minimally invasive Le Fort I with patient specific implants. Proof of concept. J Stomatol Oral Maxillofac Surf. 2024;125:101844.

10 Minimally Invasive Surgery of the Mandible

Adaia Valls Ontañón
and Federico Hernández-Alfaro

10.1 Introduction

Bilateral sagittal split ramus osteotomy (BSSO) is widely used in orthognathic surgery for the correction of mandibular deformities [1, 2]. It offers advantages over other mandibular osteotomies due to the wide overlapping cutting surface, which enables a variable range of three-dimensional (3D) movements of the distal segment, ensuring broad enough surface contact for osteosynthesis and bone healing [3].

The technique was originally introduced by Trauner and Obwegeser in 1955 [4, 5], with two horizontal cortical cuts being made along the lateral oblique ridge (one cut at the inner cortex above the Spix spine and another in the outer cortex at the gonial angle), followed by connection with chiseling. Thus, the inferior alveolar nerve (IAN) was not damaged. The cortical cuts had a distance of at least 25 mm in order to mobilize the distal segment while overlapping both bony segments. The original technique has undergone a number of modifications since the original description [6] in order to reduce complications and expand the indications. In particular, mention should be made of the modifications introduced by Dal Pont in 1961 [7] and Epker in 1977 [8]. Dal Pont [7] suggested running the osteotomy forward, taking it along the mandibular body to the level of the second and first molars, where it descended vertically to the basilar rim. In this way, the contact surface was increased, which improved bone healing and gave the technique greater versatility, allowing larger ranges of sagittal and rotational movements. In turn, Epker [8] proposed performing the osteotomy without reaching the posterior edge of the mandibular ramus but only extending up to the upper posterior area of the Spix spine, allowing a direct and careful visualization of the dental nerve, making surgical fracture more predictable, and significantly shortening the surgical time.

When performed in the context of bimaxillary surgery, in the protocol of the authors, the mandible is operated first (except when maxillary patient-specific implants are used). There are two main reasons for this approach. First, most of our patients require counterclockwise rotational movements of the maxillomandibular complex. In this scenario, operating the maxilla first would require a huge wedge-shaped intermediate splint. It would be difficult to install, and an excessive posterior rotation of the proximal (condylar fragment) would be required (Fig. 10.1) [9]. Second, since we incorporated 3D planning and CAD/CAM splints in our practice in 2010, we realized that any error in capturing the mandibular position in cone-beam computed tomography (CBCT) would imply mispositioning of the

A. Valls Ontañón (✉) · F. Hernández-Alfaro
Department of Oral and Maxillofacial Surgery, International University of Catalonia, Barcelona, Spain
e-mail: avalls@uic.es; h.alfaro@uic.es

F. Hernández-Alfaro, A. Valls Ontañón (eds.), *Orthofacial Surgery*,
https://doi.org/10.1007/978-3-031-76185-0_10

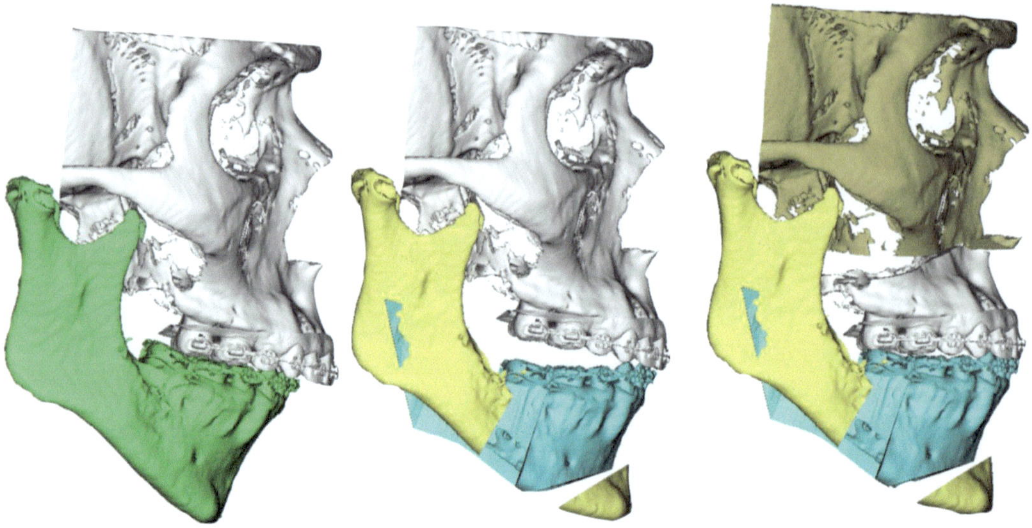

Fig. 10.1 Virtual surgical planning following the "mandible first" protocol in a case with maxillomandibular complex counterclockwise rotation. In such a scenario, the "maxillary first" protocol would require a wedge-shaped intermediate splint

maxilla if we followed the "maxilla first" protocol [10]. If this same situation were to occur in the "mandible first" protocol, the error would be "absorbed" at the level of the osteotomy and would not be translated into the distal fragment of the mandible.

The surgery is performed under general anesthesia; although when monomandibular surgery is carried out by an experienced surgeon, it could be performed under local anesthesia and sedation. Even in procedures under general anesthesia, infiltration is made with saline solution, adrenaline, and lidocaine in order to minimize bleeding and reduce the pain signals sent from the peripheral nerves to the brain, thereby lowering the general anesthetic requirements.

10.2 Surgical Approach

- The surgical *incision* is drawn over the external oblique mandibular ridge from the middle of the mandibular ramus to the level of the second molar, leaving enough nonkeratinized mucosa over the incision for posterior suturing. The use of an electric scalpel can simultaneously cut mucosa, muscle, and periosteum.
- When concomitant *extraction of an erupted or partially erupted wisdom tooth* is required, the incision should be modified in order to include keratinized mucosa surrounding the wisdom tooth for total closure of the wound at the end of the surgery (Fig. 10.2). However, our preference is to remove third molars at least 6 months before skeletal surgery.
- *Subperiosteal dissection* is mandatory to avoid hemorrhage and damage to the surrounding soft tissues. It starts in the oblique line, and on the buccal side, it should cover the area between the first molar and the lower insertions of the temporalis muscle in the anterior aspect of the ascending ramus, which allows for a better view of the surgical field. The inferior border of the mandibular body only needs to be dissected in the area where the vertical osteotomy will be placed.
- Special attention should be paid to *avoid periosteal perforation* when subperiosteal dissection of the *lingual cortex* is carried out, in order to avoid hemorrhage and lingual nerve damage. The periosteum is elevated from top to bottom until the lingula and the

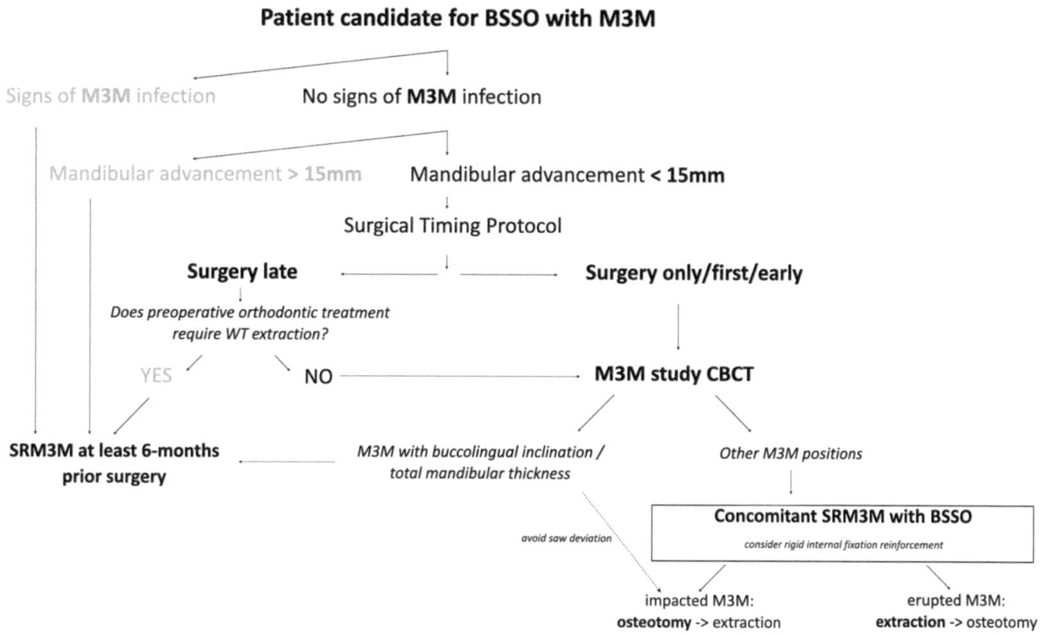

Fig. 10.2 Decision-making algorithm for concomitant mandibular third molar surgical removal with bilateral sagittal split osteotomy

neuromuscular bundle entering the mandible are found. The authors prefer lingual nerve or lingula visualization instead of placing a hook into the Spix spine, since even when performed gently, it could damage the nerve. Similarly, the authors do not use the Obwegeser retractor in this area in order to avoid excessive pressure on the bundle. Instead, the periosteal elevator is left in place, protecting the neurovascular bundle with light tension.

10.3 Osteotomy

The sagittal osteotomy design implies the initial cut of four cortical bony lines or sections which then must be completed by chiseling: horizontally through the lingual cortex, longitudinally through the mandibular ramus and lateral oblique ridge of the body, and vertically through the buccal cortex, followed by the lower basal border. To avoid a bad-split fracture, all of the cortex must be completely traversed and the bone marrow reached. Regarding the cutting tools, although the authors use a reciprocating saw with a thin blade (2 cm long and 1.5 mm thick), some surgeons feel more comfortable using a Lindeman burr or a piezoelectric device.

- First section: *Lingual cortex osteotomy*. After lingual nerve visualization and protection, the sagittal osteotomy starts from the lingual cortical cut, which should be parallel to the occlusal plane. A beveled cut is initiated just over the bundle. It is of utmost importance to stay within 5 mm over the entrance of the lingula, as going further up implies entering the risk zone where the lingual and buccal plates are fused and a bad split can easily happen (Fig. 10.3). It is also important to make sure that it posteriorly overtakes the lingula [11, 12].
- Second section: *Longitudinal osteotomy over the ridge*. The connection between the first and second sections of the osteotomy should have a smooth “S” pattern, avoiding angles which could later facilitate bad splits. By looking at the CBCT, one can easily understand the 3D position of the bundle and design

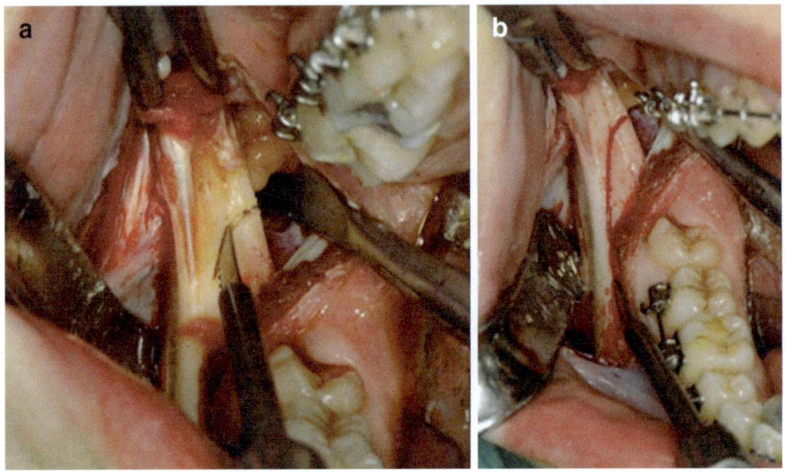

Fig. 10.3 Intraoperative view showing first (**a**) and second (**b**) sections of the mandibular sagittal osteotomy, where the beveled cut is initiated just over the lingual bundle and right angles are avoided

the pattern of the osteotomy accordingly (Fig. 10.3). The authors recommend not penetrating more than 5–10 mm (according to the preoperative CBCT measurements) with the blade and staying 5 mm lingual to the buccal wall (or just medial to the buccal cortex) in order to avoid damage to the nerve. It is performed from top to bottom and usually ends medial to the second molar, though it might be expanded when large advancements and/or counterclockwise rotations are required. The tip of the saw should always be parallel to the buccal wall to avoid crossing it again due to the inward curve of the mandibular angle shape.

  – In the event of an impacted wisdom tooth, its hardness may complicate the osteotomy, and special attention should be paid to avoid saw deviation (Fig. 10.2).

- Third section: *Vertical or mesial osteotomy*. This is usually placed medial to the second molar, though it might be expanded when large advancements and/or counterclockwise rotations are required. The authors recommend performing the buccal osteotomy running backward to the posterior limit of the antegonial notch instead of a vertical osteotomy, in order to reduce the gap in the buccal osteotomy (Fig. 10.4). Again, the vertical cut should not penetrate more than 5 mm on the cortical plate. To protect the buccal and submandibular soft tissues, an Obwegeser retractor is used (Fig. 10.5).

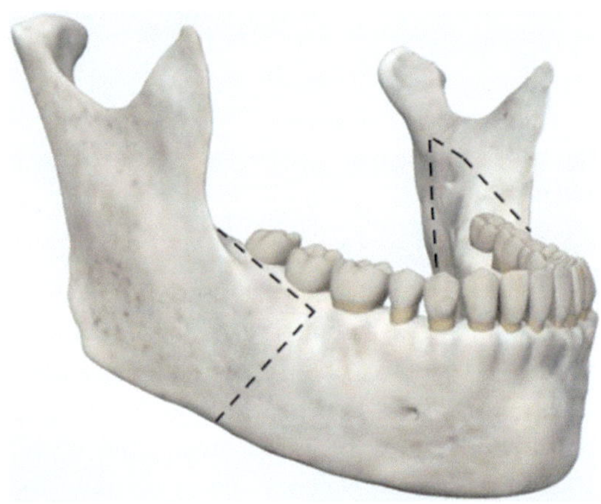

Fig. 10.4 View showing backward direction of the vertical buccal osteotomy (third section) to the antegonial notch in order to reduce the buccal gap

- Fourth section: *Inferior mandibular border osteotomy*. This is the most common source of bad splits, according to the literature [13, 14]. With the patient's mouth closed and protection provided by the Obwegeser retractor, a down-to-up cut is made. It is imperative to completely cut all the basal thickness of the mandibular body; otherwise, when performing the split, the border will remain attached to the anterior fragment, and this will automatically provoke a bad split.

- For chiseling purposes, the authors mostly use a 10 mm osteotome, although plenty of osteotomes have been described for this maneuver [3, 15]. The osteotomes should not be inserted more than 5–10 mm (depending on the patient anatomy), in order to avoid inferior alveolar nerve damage. When malleting the osteotome, the mandibular body should be held in order to avoid edema or hemarthrosis of the temporomandibular joint.

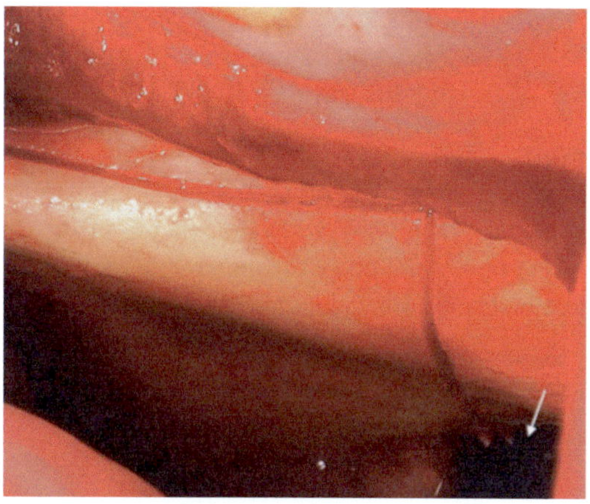

Fig. 10.5 Third and fourth sections of the mandibular sagittal osteotomy using an Obwegeser retractor (arrow) to protect the buccal and submandibular soft tissues

- The authors separate both segments with a 10 mm wedge-shaped osteotome malleted exactly at the connection between the upper and longitudinal cuts (first and second sections). This initiates separation of the plates. Then, the Smith ramus separator is inserted at the longitudinal (second) section of the osteotomy. Simultaneous twisting of the osteotome and opening the spreader allows for a gentle separation of the plates and location of the bundle (Fig. 10.6). This maneuver should not require much force. If too much resistance is noted, the osteotomies should be rechecked (especially the fourth section).
- Occasionally, when performing the actual split, we can find the bundle attached to the buccal plate (proximal or condylar fragment). With the aid of a small spatula and/or piezoelectric saw, we must gently detach and free it.
- Knife-edge borders of the mandibular channel may frequently arise, which might eventually damage the nerve after the proximal fragment

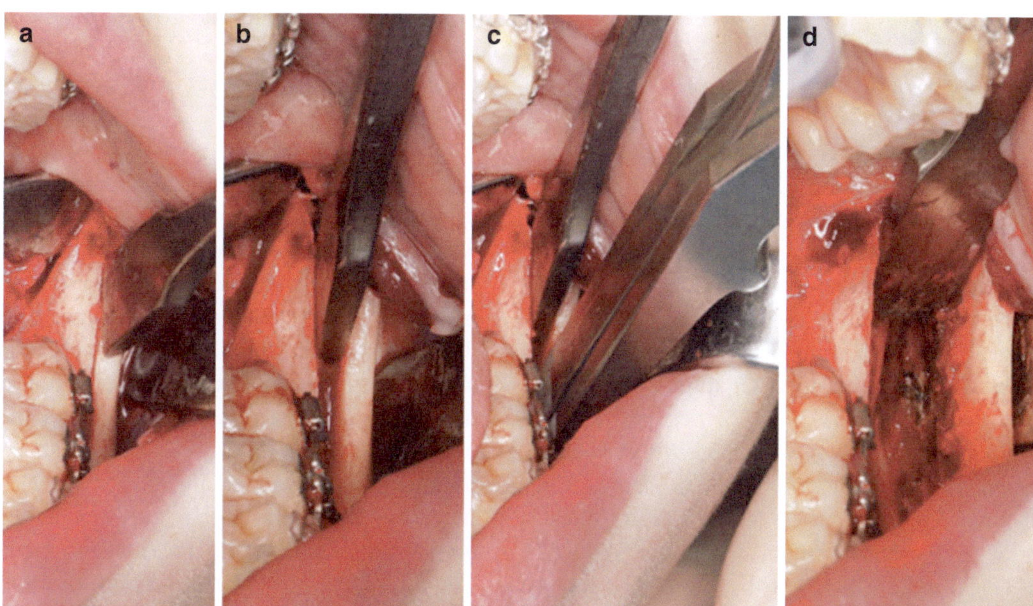

Fig. 10.6 Intraoperative view showing separation of both segments with the 10 mm osteotome placed posteriorly (**a**), which is slightly opened (**b**) to introduce the Smith ramus separator anteriorly (**c**), and the split is completed with both tools at the same time under direct visualization to control the position of the inferior alveolar nerve (**d**)

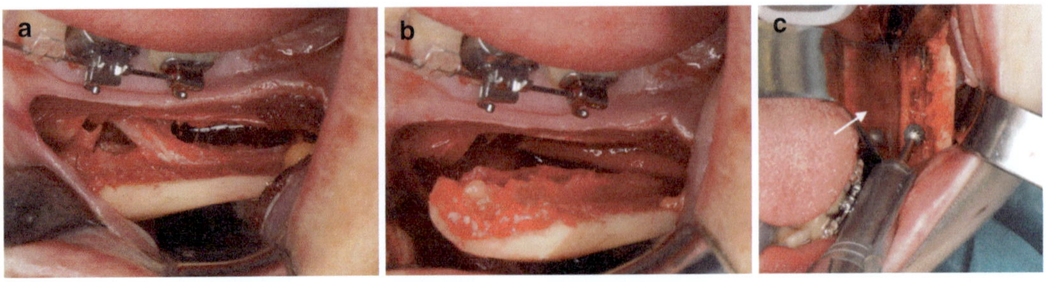

Fig. 10.7 After inferior alveolar nerve detachment from the proximal segment (**a**), bone spicules may arise (**b**), which should be removed while protecting the nerve (arrow) to avoid inferior alveolar nerve damage after mandibular repositioning (**c**)

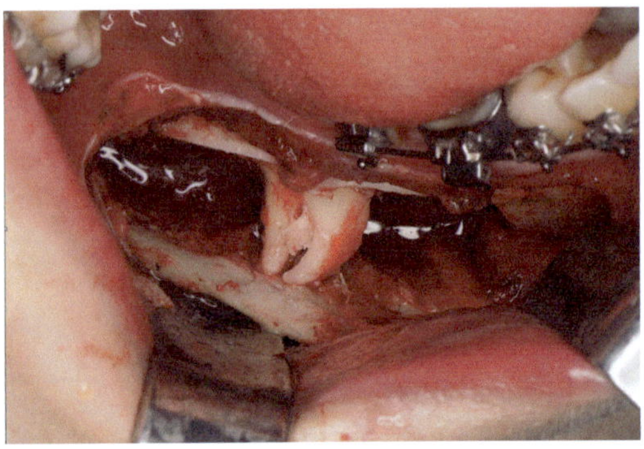

Fig. 10.8 Impacted wisdom teeth are removed after completing the sagittal split separation in order to avoid extra bone removal and allow better visualization of the surgical field

is repositioned. To avoid this, we can use a burr or the piezo inset to smoothen the inner surface of the lateral plate (Fig. 10.7).

- After completing the separation, proper separation from the pterygomasseteric sling should be ensured in order to allow proper 3D mobilization of both segments.
- In cases where an impacted third molar needs to be extracted, it should be performed after complete separation and under direct visualization of the inferior alveolar nerve. The approach is thus easier, and the risk of damage to the neurovascular bundle is reduced (Figs. 10.2 and 10.8) [16].

Customized cutting guides for BSSO are not recommended because they do not afford enough precision of the deeper cutting area of the tip of the saw, which may produce deviation of the tip of the saw in the deeper plane and therefore lead to a bad split [10, 17].

10.4 Condylar or Proximal Segment Positioning and Osteosynthesis

Proper intraoperative proximal segment positioning entails 3D evaluation and involves several factors such as bony interferences, condyle settlement, muscular pulling, and the type of osteosynthesis, among others [18]. Thus, the authors recommend the following key points to ensure proper positioning:

- Intermaxillary fixation with the intermediate splint in place and fixed with at least three wire loops: one anterior and two posterior.
- Interferences between the distal and proximal bony segments precluding gentle settlement of the proximal segment should be checked, since they may lead to external shifting of the proximal segment and taking the condyle out of the fossa (Fig. 10.9) [19]. If there is any interference, it should be milled.
- In cases where the lingula does not allow proper settlement of the proximal segment (such as large mandibular advancement or centering), a greenstick osteotomy of the lingual cortical layer of the distal segment should be performed with a piezoelectric saw (also called lingual osteotomy), without stripping

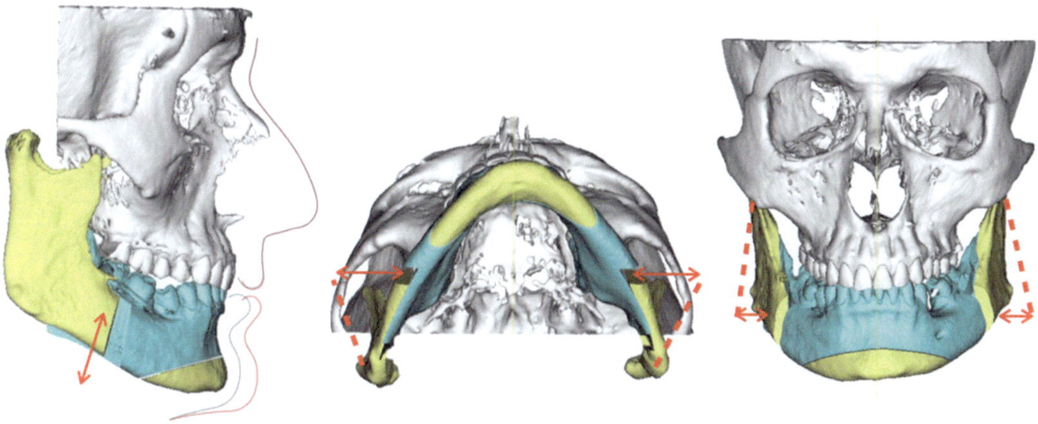

Fig. 10.9 Three-dimensional settlement of the mandibular proximal segments in order to avoid mismatches between distal and proximal fragments is shown in the virtual orthognathic surgery planning

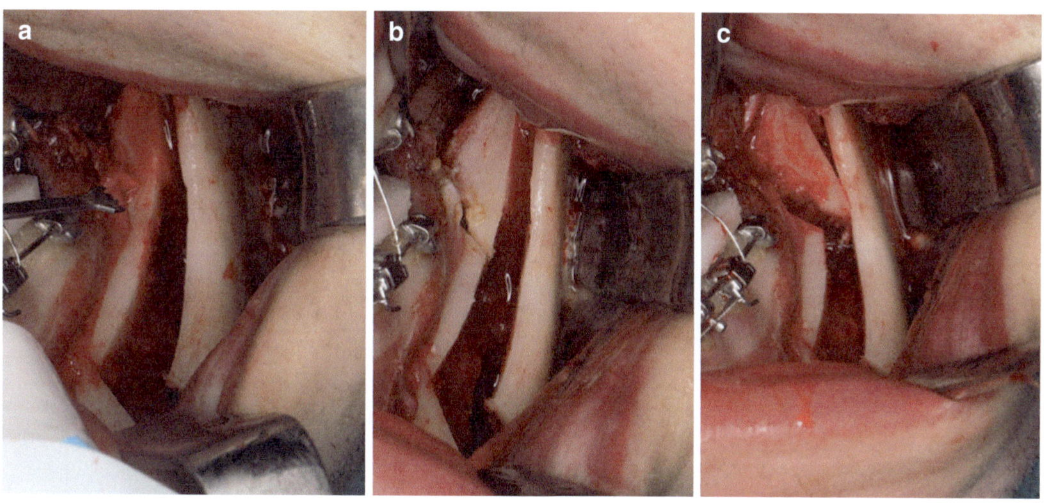

Fig. 10.10 Intraoperative views showing (**a**) interference between the distal segment and left proximal segment; (**b**) lingual osteotomy; and (**c**) smooth transition between the left proximal and distal segments after lingual osteotomy. Note that the osteotomized bone fragment is left in place

the soft tissues on the lingual surface, and leaving the osteotomized bone fragment in place in order to avoid nerve damage (Fig. 10.10). This technique should enable smooth transition between the segments and proper 3D repositioning of the distal segment with passive accommodation of the condyle at the glenoid fossa, while increasing the contact surface between the two fragments [12].

- Then, Kocher forceps are used to grasp the proximal fragment, and the appropriate mini-plate is fixed in it with two monocortical screws (Fig. 10.11).
- For vertical and sagittal condylar positioning, several devices have been described, but they are too time-consuming, difficult to use, and most importantly, there is no evidence of better results than with manual positioning [20]. Thus, the authors recommend manual positioning of the proximal segment. As a routine measure, proper seating of the condyles into the uppermost anterior part of the fossa should

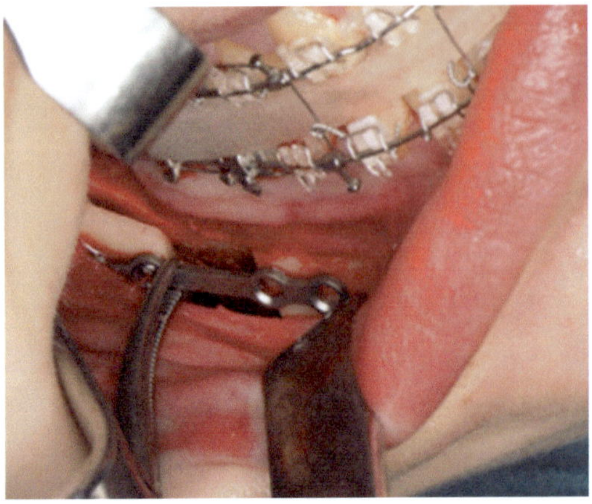

Fig. 10.11 Proper settlement and fixation of the proximal segment

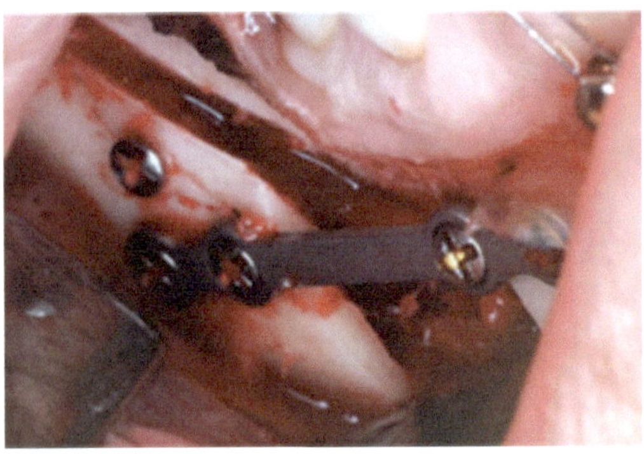

Fig. 10.12 Intraoperative view showing mandibular rigid internal fixation after BSSO using a hybrid technique: a mini-plate fixed with four monocortical screws and a retromolar bicortical screw

be ensured with a bidirectional maneuver, applying two force vectors: one hand gently repositions the condylar segment posteriorly, while the other hand is used to push up and forward the mandibular angle extraorally, thus allowing proper settlement of the condyle in the anterior uppermost point of the glenoid fossa [20].

- After proper condylar positioning, the anterior portion of the plate is fixed to the distal fragment with two additional monocortical screws.
- Then, a retromolar bicortical screw is placed to complete the rigid internal fixation hybrid technique (Fig. 10.12). Placing a mini-plate fixed with four monocortical screws and a retromolar bicortical screw is advised, since it provides enough stability while allowing proper condyle accommodation to the glenoid fossa [3]. When introducing the bicortical screw, it is mandatory to take care that the initial gap between both segments is maintained, otherwise it might lead to a medial shift of the condyle.
  - When a "mandible first" protocol is chosen, we need to have rigid fixation on the mandible by means of the hybrid technique, which will act as the template on top of which a semirigidly fixed maxilla will be placed.
  - In monomandibular surgeries, a single mini-plate with four monocortical screws provides enough stability, since maxillary steadiness reinforces that of the mandible.
  - On the other hand, rigid fixation is reinforced with two mini-plates in the following situations: large advancement (>2 cm), concomitant wisdom tooth extraction leaving a sizeable bone gap, and lingula osteotomy that does not allow enough room for retromolar bicortical screw placement.
- Finally, the intermaxillary fixation is removed, and before removing the intermediate splint, proper condylar positioning and intermediate occlusion are checked by passive adjustment of the mandible into the splint.
- Placing a gauze embedded in hydrogen peroxide on each side during the rest of the surgery is recommended in order to control any residual oozing.

It is important to highlight that after orthognathic surgery, the condylar shape may change or remodel secondary to condyle accommodation to new anatomic skeletal changes and muscle function. These functional changes do not imply temporomandibular joint pathology, however [21].

10.5 Suturing and Closure

Wound irrigation to remove any debris is recommended before surgical closure. Suture should grab periosteum, muscle, and mucosa in the flap

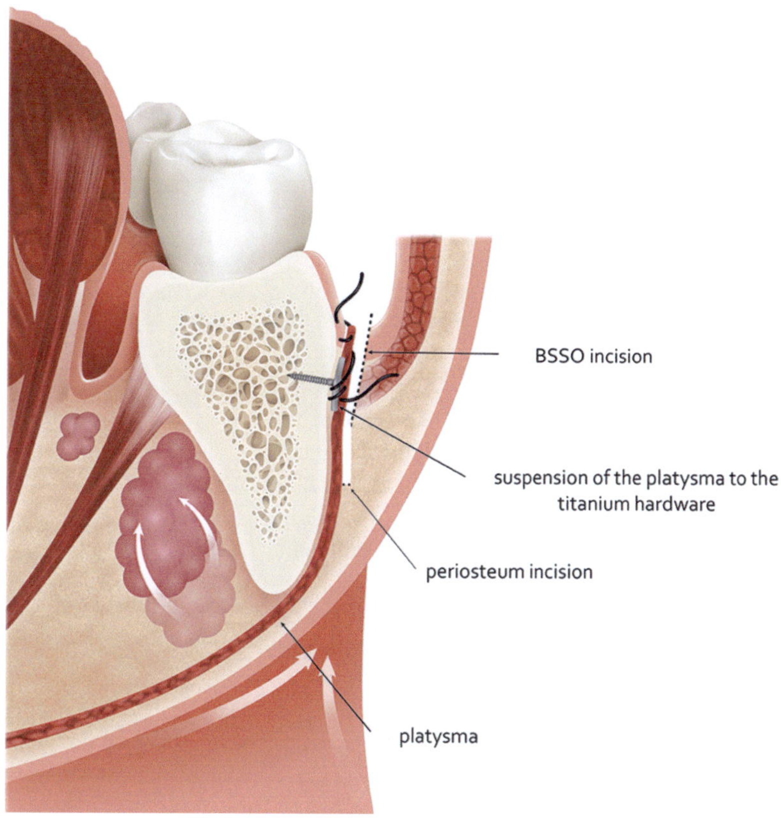

Fig. 10.13 Schematic view showing the technique used for suspension of the platysma of the upper aspect of the submandibular space

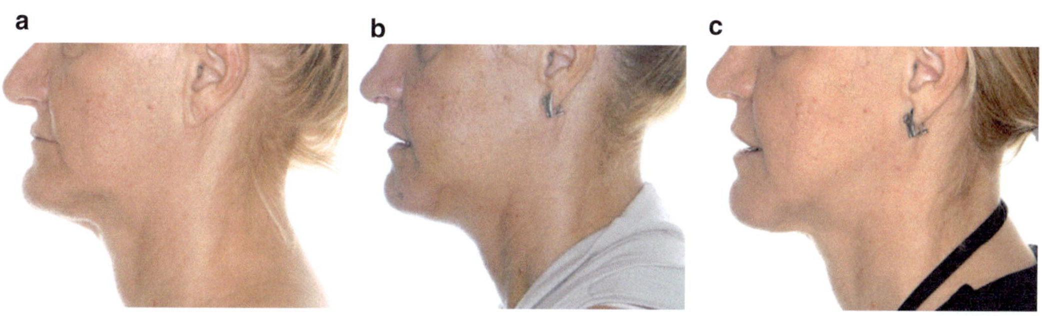

Fig. 10.14 Preoperative (**a**) and postoperative views illustrating the short- (1 month) (**b**) and long-term (6 months) (**c**) effect of the intraoral neck lift

to ensure adequate repositioning of the soft tissues.

Some elderly patients present with a visible bulge in the area of the submandibular salivary gland that disrupts the flat and smooth surface of a youthful appearing neck. Therefore, suspension of the platysma of the upper aspect of the submandibular space to the uppermost mandibular periosteum or osteosynthesis hardware through the BSSO approach can be performed to improve the jawline contour and produce a neck rejuvenating effect (Figs. 10.13 and 10.14) [11].

10.6 Key Points

- The mandible is operated first in most cases.
- When monomandibular surgery is carried out by an experienced surgeon, it could be performed under local anesthesia and sedation.
- Customized cutting guides for BSSO are not recommended.
- Proper subperiosteal dissection avoids hemorrhage and provides good visualization of the surgical field, apart from avoiding nerve damage.
- A proper cortex cut reaching the bone marrow of the sagittal osteotomy including lingual cortex, mandibular ramus and lateral oblique ridge of the body, and buccal cortex including the inferior basal border avoids a bad-split fracture.
- When chiseling, the osteotomes should not be inserted more than 5 mm in order to avoid inferior alveolar nerve damage.
- Separation of both segments is carried out under direct visualization of proper separation of the two segments and inferior alveolar nerve preservation.
- Interferences between the distal and proximal bony segments should be checked for proper condyle settlement.
- Proper seating of the condyles into the uppermost anterior part of the fossa should be ensured with a bidirectional maneuver.
- Rigid internal fixation using a hybrid technique (a mini-plate fixed with four monocortical screws and a retromolar bicortical screw) is recommended, since it provides enough stability while allowing proper condyle accommodation to the glenoid fossa.
- Suspension of the platysma of the upper aspect of the submandibular space to the uppermost mandibular periosteum can be performed to improve the jawline contour.

References

1. Obwegeser H. The indications for surgical correction of mandibular deformity by the sagittal splitting technique. Br J Oral Surg. 1963;1(C):157–71.
2. Wolford LM, Bennett MA, Rafferty CG. Modification of the mandibular ramus sagittal split osteotomy. Oral Surg Oral Med Oral Pathol. 1987;64(2):146–55.
3. Hernández-Alfaro F, Raffaini M, Paredes-de-Sousa-Gil A, Magri AS, Guijarro-Martínez R, Valls-Ontañón A. Three-dimensional analysis of long-term stability after bilateral sagittal Split ramus osteotomy fixed with a single miniplate with 4 monocortical screws and 1 bicortical screw: a retrospective 2-center study. J Oral Maxillofac Surg. 2017;75(5):1036–45.
4. Trauner R, Obwegeser H. The surgical correction of mandibular prognathism and retrognathia with consideration of genioplasty. II. Operating methods for microgenia and distoclusion. Oral Surg Oral Med Oral Pathol. 1957;10(9):899–909.
5. Trauner R, Obwegeser H. The surgical correction of mandibular prognathism and retrognathia with consideration of genioplasty. I. Surgical procedures to correct mandibular prognathism and reshaping of the chin. Oral Surg Oral Med Oral Pathol. 1957;10(7):677–89.
6. Böckmann R, Meyns J, Dik E, Kessler P. The modifications of the sagittal ramus split osteotomy: a literature review. Plast Reconstr Surg Glob Open. 2014;2(12):e271.
7. Dal Pont G. Retromolar osteotomy for the correction of prognathism. J Oral Surg Anesth Hosp Dent Serv. 1961 Jan;19:42–7.
8. Epker BN. Modifications in the sagittal osteotomy of the mandible. J Oral Surg. 1977;35(2):157–9.
9. Perez D, Ellis E III. Sequencing bimaxillary surgery: mandible first. YJOMS [Internet]. 2011;69(8):2217–24. https://doi.org/10.1016/j.joms.2010.10.053.
10. Aboul-Hosn Centenero S, Hernández-Alfaro F. 3D planning in orthognathic surgery: CAD/CAM surgical splints and prediction of the soft and hard tissues results—our experience in 16 cases. J Cranio-Maxillofac Surg. 2012;40(2):162–8.
11. Hernández-Alfaro F, Guijarro-Martínez R, Masià-Gridilla J, Valls-Ontañón A. Jawline contouring through an intraoral approach in the context of bilateral sagittal Split osteotomy: a proof-of-concept report. J Oral Maxillofac Surg. 2019;77(1):174–8.
12. Valls-Ontañón A, Ascencio-Padilla RDJ, Vela-Lasagabaster A, Sada-Malumbres A, Haas-Junior OL,

Masià-Gridilla J, et al. Relevance of 3D virtual planning in predicting bony interferences between distal and proximal fragments after sagittal split osteotomy. Int J Oral Maxillofac Surg. 2020;49(8):1020–8.

13. Houppermans PNWJ, Verweij JP, Mensink G, Gooris PJJ, van Merkesteyn JPR. Influence of inferior border cut on lingual fracture pattern during bilateral sagittal split osteotomy with splitter and separators: a prospective observational study. J Cranio-Maxillofac Surg. 2016;44(10):1592–8.
14. Steenen SA, van Wijk AJ, Becking AG. Bad splits in bilateral sagittal split osteotomy: systematic review and meta-analysis of reported risk factors. Int J Oral Maxillofac Surg. 2016;45(8):971–9.
15. Raffaini M, Hernandez Alfaro F, Ghilardi R, Garcia LA. The sagittal mandibular osteotomy under local anesthesia and intravenous sedation: four years of multicenter experience. Int J Adult Orthodon Orthognath Surg. 2002;17(4):267–71.
16. Doucet JC, Morrison AD, Davis BR, Gregoire CE, Goodday R, Precious DS. The presence of mandibular third molars during sagittal split osteotomies does not increase the risk of complications. YJOMS [Internet]. 2012;70(8):1935–43. https://doi.org/10.1016/j.joms.2011.08.018.
17. Philippe B. Accuracy of position of cutting and drilling guide for sagittal split guided surgery: a proof of concept study. Br J Oral Maxillofac Surg [Internet]. 2020;58:940. https://doi.org/10.1016/j.bjoms.2020.04.034.
18. Méndez-Manjón I, Guijarro-Martínez R, Valls-Otañón A, Hernandez-Alfaro F. Early changes in condylar position after mandibular advancement: a three-dimensional analysis. Int J Oral Maxillofac Surg. 2016;45:787–92.
19. Reyneke JP, Ferretti C. Intraoperative diagnosis of condylar sag after bilateral sagittal split ramus osteotomy. Br J Oral Maxillofac Surg. 2002;4356:285–92.
20. Costa F, Robiony M, Toro C, Sembronio S, Polini F, Politi M. Condylar positioning devices for orthognathic surgery: a literature review, vol. 106; 2008. p. 179.
21. Mendez-Manjon I, Guijarro-Martinez R, Valls-Ontañón A, Hernandez-Alfaro F. Early changes in condylar position after mandibular advancement: a three-dimensional analysis. Int J Oral Maxillofac Surg. 2016;45(6):787–92.

Surgery of the Chin

11

Adaia Valls Ontañón
and Federico Hernández-Alfaro

11.1 Introduction

The chin makes a fundamental contribution to facial aesthetics. This anterior part of the mandible can present structural and/or positional problems. An appropriate chin position and proportion results in an adequate lip–chin relationship, contributes to normal vertical proportions, and gives support to the submandibular soft tissues [1].

In most instances, appropriate repositioning of the mandible can normalize the three-dimensional (3D) chin projection [2]. However, there are a number of circumstances in which the chin needs to be independently repositioned or reshaped in order to achieve an adequate aesthetic balance in the lower facial third. Genioplasty is a surgical procedure that allows correction of chin dimensions and asymmetries. Specifically, in the sliding genioplasty procedure, the chin bone (symphysis and parasymphysis) is moved three-dimensionally to a planned position to improve the facial aesthetic appearance or correct an eventual asymmetry [2].

Genioplasty was first described by Hofer in 1952 [3] and was popularized by Converse and Wood-Smith in 1964 [4]. Since then, the procedure has developed as a versatile technique to correct both deficient and excessive chin deformities.

The procedure may be performed in the context of orthognathic surgery or as a sole procedure. In the latter case, it could be performed under local anesthesia and sedation. When genioplasty is carried out in the context of "trimaxillary" surgery, it is advisable to perform it after maxillary and mandibular repositioning and leaving the intermaxillary fixation in place, which ties up the mandible and therefore eases the procedure [2, 5]. Even under general anesthesia, infiltration is made with saline solution, adrenaline, and lidocaine in order to minimize bleeding and reduce the pain signals sent from the peripheral nerves to the brain, thus reducing the general anesthetic needs.

Chin contouring without osteotomies is rarely indicated but might have a role when minor changes in shape are needed. Small sagittal reductions and small asymmetries might benefit from this "ostectomy" approach.

On the other hand, we do not advocate prosthetic chin augmentation for two basic reasons. First, chin prosthesis effects are basically limited to anteroposterior augmentation. Second, over time, there is a tendency to penetrate the underlying bone, thus provoking a loss of chin projection and altering the morphology of the chin itself and of the surrounding soft tissues. We have rarely applied chin prostheses (some syndromic cases with a lack of bone stock) but have removed

A. Valls Ontañón (✉) · F. Hernández-Alfaro
Department of Oral and Maxillofacial Surgery, International University of Catalonia, Barcelona, Spain
e-mail: avalls@uic.es; h.alfaro@uic.es

F. Hernández-Alfaro, A. Valls Ontañón (eds.), *Orthofacial Surgery*,
https://doi.org/10.1007/978-3-031-76185-0_11

dozens of them. Exceptionally, in cases of major reconstruction of congenital, oncological, or traumatologic anomalies, prostheses may be considered as an option.

11.2 Surgical Planning

Chin surgery assessment requires a complete facial analysis and specific evaluation of the lower third, taking into consideration the dental relationship, maxillomandibular skeletal morphology, and the soft-tissue envelope [6].

Although individual patient preferences need to be taken into account, the following aesthetic principles of the area are helpful for chin surgery planning:

- Chin *asymmetries* may be assessed.
- *Transverse* dimension: Males tend to have a square, wider (interpupillary length), and more projected chin that may have a two-point light reflection. Females, on the other hand, tend to have a narrower chin (intercanthal length) with a single-point light reflection [7].
- The *vertical* dimension is variable depending on the ethnicity: The height of the lower third of the face should be equal to that of the upper and middle thirds. Furthermore, lower facial height is in turn divided into an upper third (upper lip) and two lower thirds (lower lip and chin). An increased incisor display and/or mentalis strain/lip incompetence can indicate a long-face growth pattern (Fig. 11.1), whereas a decreased incisor display can signal a short-face growth pattern [8].
- The *sagittal* projection of the chin should never project beyond the Riedel line [7], although our reference is to trace a rectangular angle between the bony chin and the occlusal plane in the sagittal view (Fig. 11.2). Besides, a proper labiomental fold should be considered, being approximately 4 mm in males and 6 mm in women [9], though this also depends on the underlying dental support [10].

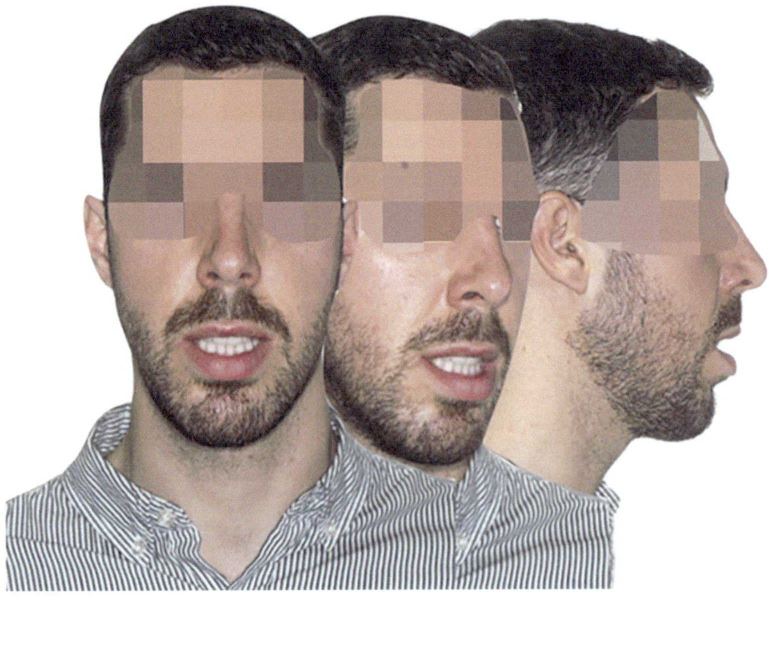

Fig. 11.1 Increased incisor display and/or mentalis strain/lip incompetence can indicate a vertical and/or sagittal chin anomaly

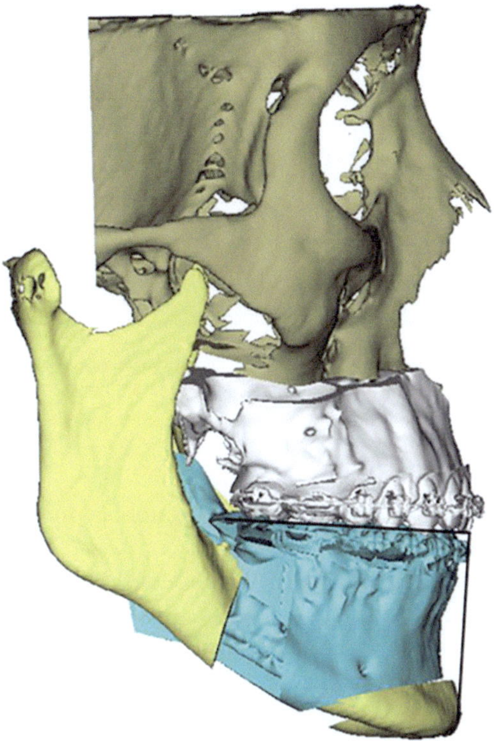

Fig. 11.2 Surgical planning sagittal reference: rectangular angle between the bony chin and the occlusal plane

11.3 Surgical Approach

The conventional approach comprises a horizontal incision 5 mm below the keratinized mucosa and between the two canines. The incision is carried down through the mucosa, mentalis muscle, and periosteum, leaving a generous cuff of mucosa and muscle that will allow for a tight closure. Our choice is to use an electrical scalpel with a fine tip. Although subperiosteal dissection should be limited to the osteotomy line and area of osteosynthesis placement, localization of the mental foramen and dental roots is recommended in order to avoid mental nerve and root damage, respectively. It is important to avoid extensive dissection, as the soft-tissue attachments help to stabilize the skeletal alteration, minimize unpredictable soft-tissue changes, and lessen postoperative bone resorption [11, 12].

Recently, a minimally invasive vertical incision has been described [13], in which a short vertical incision is made through the lower lip frenulum, below the mucogingival junction. Then, a sharp incision is made through the periosteum at the midline, and subperiosteal dissection is performed under the mentalis muscles without the release or transection of the latter, toward the lower mandibular border. The mentalis muscles are kept intact, eliminating possible muscle dysfunctions [13].

11.4 Osteotomy

The chin osteotomy can be made with a reciprocating saw, Lindeman burr, or piezoelectric saw. The first step is to mark three reference lines above and below the osteotomy line: one at the interincisal midline and two at the laterals. They might be helpful for 3D symmetric repositioning of the distal segment of the chin to match the facial midline [6, 13].

Then, the chin osteotomy is drawn according to the surgical planning and at least 5 mm below the mental foramens and roots of the canines. Every effort should be made to perform symmetrical osteotomies on both sides (unless dealing with an asymmetrical chin). In general terms, the more posteriorly the osteotomy is extended, the better. This will minimize the step between the lower border of the mandible and the mobilized chin, thus favoring a smoother transition. However, in female patients, the osteotomy is rhomboid shaped in order to not widen the chin.

It is important to make complete cuts, i.e., along both the anterior buccal and posterior lingual cortex in order to avoid an incomplete osteotomy. The inclination of the saw will determine the direction of sliding and thus the final position of the distal segment:

- A *horizontal osteotomy* will lead to pure advancement of the chin and therefore chin height maintenance (Fig. 11.3).
- A *more upright osteotomy* will lead to upward advancement of the chin and therefore chin height reduction (Fig. 11.3).

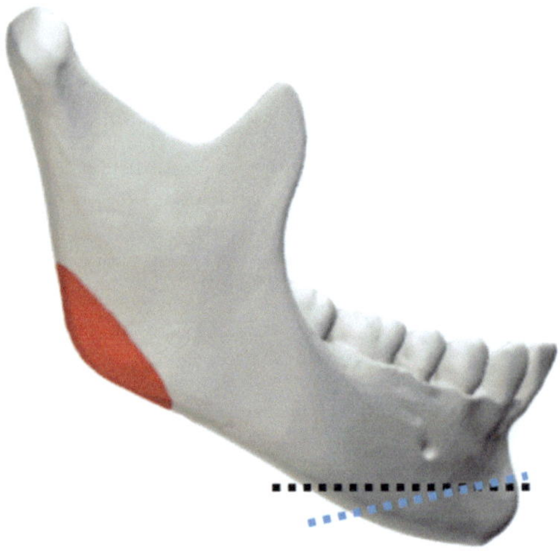

Fig. 11.3 The inclination of the saw will determine the direction of sliding and thus the final positioning of the distal segment. While a horizontal osteotomy will lead to pure advancement of the chin (black dotted line), a more upright osteotomy will lead to upward advancement of the chin (blue dotted line)

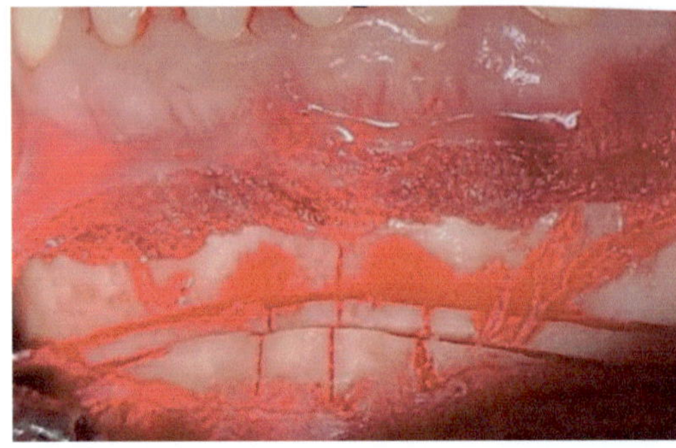

Fig. 11.4 Intraoperative view showing two parallel osteotomies to take out a bony slice for chin height reduction. Note the three reference lines above and below the osteotomy line

When required, the osteotomy may be completed with an osteotome. Distal segment mobilization might be jeopardized by suprahyoid muscles, which eventually must be partially elongated. Sharp edges of bone should be reshaped, as well as bony interferences.

On the other hand, beside sagittal movements (vertical and anteroposterior), the chin can also be rotated with roll, yaw, and pitch movements. We rarely consider posterior chin repositioning, since this might have a negative impact upon the submandibular tissues and provoke a "witch chin deformity." When excessive chin projection is associated, we favor a hinge type of rotation where the center of roll would be axial through the posterior points of the osteotomy. This is typically indicated in short faces.

For height reduction purposes with proper or too much chin projection, a second parallel osteotomy should be performed and a bony slice taken out (Fig. 11.4). When modification of the transverse dimension of the chin is planned, a vertical osteotomy should be performed for both widening or narrowing purposes.

Finally, although it is a routine and simple procedure, obtaining a symmetrical osteotomy of the right and left sides of the chin might prove challenging, in the same way as positioning the distal segment properly, which might affect the symmetry of the chin at the final outcome [14]. Thus, some authors advocate the use of a customized and tooth-supported cutting and positioning guide, which can be in-house-designed and 3D-printed [15, 16].

11.5 Osteosynthesis

Rigid fixation of the chin can be carried out in two different ways. On one hand, two tricortical screws can be used, where an important tip is to bury the screw head through countersinking (Fig. 11.5). On the other hand, an X-shaped (prevent or not) mini-plate fixed with four monocortical screws can be used (Fig. 11.6). In cases of vertical augmentation of the chin, we favor the use of an X-shaped mini-plate.

When a gap remains between both segments or between the vertical osteotomes for widening purposes, an interpositional autograft, bone block allograft, or off-the-shelf material block can be placed in between (Fig. 11.7) [17].

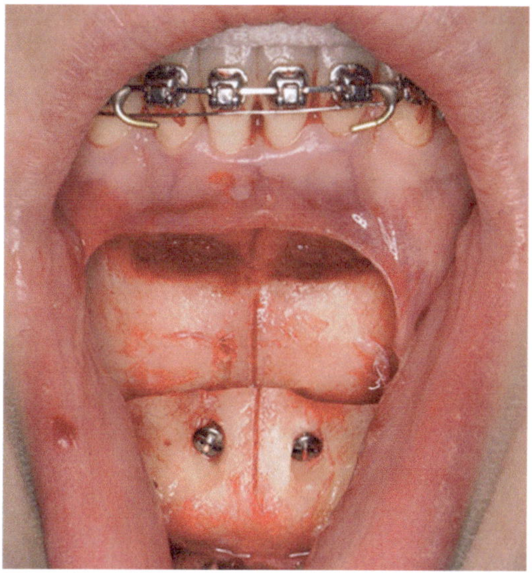

Fig. 11.5 Intraoperative view of two tricortical screws for rigid fixation. Note the buried screw head through countersinking

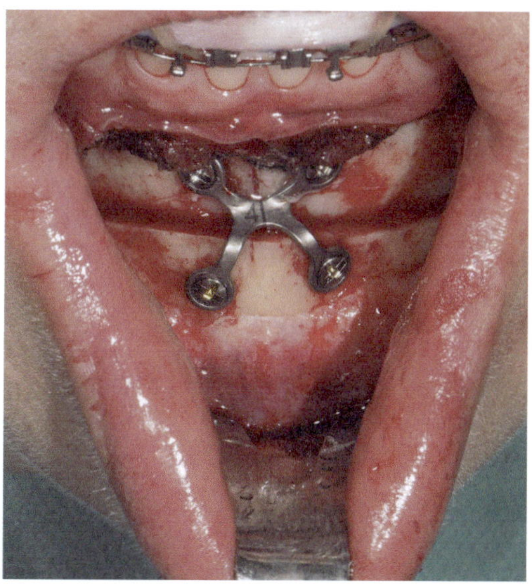

Fig. 11.6 Chin fixation with an X-shaped mini-plate (prevent) and four monocortical screws

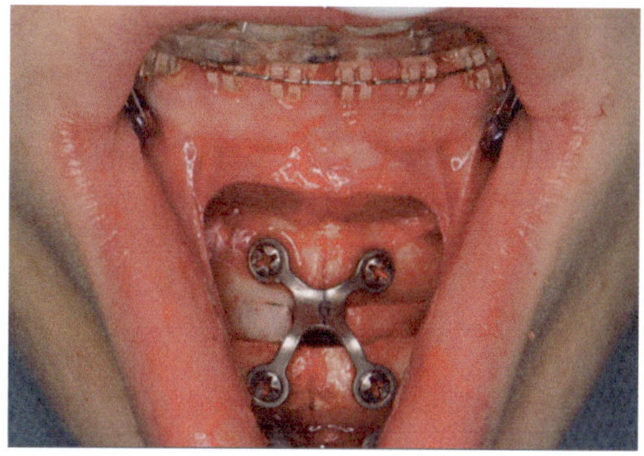

Fig. 11.7 Intraoperative view showing an interpositional autograft placed in the bony gap

11.6 Suturing and Closure

The suprahyoid muscles are repositioned by suturing them over the osteosynthesis hardware, thereby improving the neck–chin angle [18]. Thus, muscle suture should be held before placing the rigid fixation and then knotted after placing it and over it. Wound irrigation to remove any debris is recommended before surgical closure.

Then, when a conventional horizontal incision is performed, it is mandatory to resuspend the mentalis muscle to avoid a drooping chin. Finally, mucosal suturing should seal the surgical field and not damage the nerve endings of the mental nerve [19].

11.7 Key Points

- An appropriate chin position and proportion results in an adequate lip–chin relationship, contributes to normal vertical proportions, and gives support to the submandibular soft tissues.
- Prosthetic chin augmentation is not recommended as the standard genioplasty procedure.

- A minimally invasive technique preserving as much periosteum and muscle tissue as possible, and their final repositioning, is essential in order to minimize unpredictable soft-tissue changes.
- It is mandatory to avoid damage to the dental roots and mental nerve.
- The inclination of the saw will determine the direction of sliding and thus final positioning of the distal segment.
- When a gap remains between bony segments, an interpositional autograft, bone block allograft, or off-the-shelf material block can be placed in between.

References

1. Abadi M, Pour OB. Genioplasty. Facial Plast Surg. 2015;31(5):513–22.
2. Mohamed WV, Perenack JD. Aesthetic adjuncts with orthognathic surgery. Oral Maxillofac Surg Clin NA [Internet]. 2014;26:573. https://doi.org/10.1016/j.coms.2014.08.010.
3. Hofer O. [Diagnosis and therapy of the giant cell granuloma of the jaws]. Osterr Z Stomatol. 1952;49(6):324–8.
4. Converse JM, Wood-Smith D. Horizontal osteotomy of the mandible. Plast Reconstr Surg. 1964;34:464–71.
5. Storms AS, Vansant L, Shaheen E, Coucke W, de Llano-Pérula MC, Jacobs R, et al. Three-dimensional aesthetic assessment of class II patients before and after orthognathic surgery and its association with quantitative surgical changes. Int J Oral Maxillofac Surg. 2017;46(12):1664–71.
6. Lee EI. Aesthetic alteration of the chin. Semin Plast Surg. 2013;27(3):155–60.
7. Guyuron B. MOC-PS(SM) CME article: genioplasty. Plast Reconstr Surg. 2008;121(4 Suppl):1–7.
8. San Miguel Moragas J, Oth O, Büttner M, Mommaerts MY. A systematic review on soft-to-hard tissue ratios in orthognathic surgery part II: Chin procedures. J Cranio-Maxillofacial Surg [Internet]. 2015;43(8):1530–40. https://doi.org/10.1016/j.jcms.2015.07.032.
9. Zide BM, Boutros S. Chin surgery III: revelations. Plast Reconstr Surg. 2003 Apr;111(4):1542.
10. Deschamps-Braly J. Feminization of the chin: genioplasty using osteotomies. Facial Plast Surg Clin North Am [Internet]. 2019;27(2):243–50. https://doi.org/10.1016/j.fsc.2019.01.002.
11. Hoffman GR, Moloney FB. The stability of facial osteotomies. 2. Mandibular advancement with bicortical screw fixation. Aust Dent J. 1995;40(4):213–9.
12. Retana A. Controversies in facial cosmetic surgery. Oral Maxillofac Surg Clin NA [Internet]. 2017;29(4):441–6. https://doi.org/10.1016/j.coms.2017.07.002.
13. Nadjmi N, Van Roy S, Van De Casteele E. Minimally invasive genioplasty procedure. Plast Reconstr Surg-Glob Open. 2017;5(11):1–3.
14. Dong T, Ye N, Yuan L, Wu S. Assessing the influence of chin asymmetry on perceived facial esthetics with 3-dimensional images. J Oral Maxillofac Surg [Internet]. 2020;78:1–8. https://doi.org/10.1016/j.joms.2020.03.017.
15. Li B, Wei H, Zeng F, Li J, Xia JJ, Wang X. Application of a novel three-dimensional printing genioplasty template system and its clinical validation: a control study. Sci Rep [Internet]. 2017;7(1):1–8. https://doi.org/10.1038/s41598-017-05417-7.
16. Oth O, Durieux V, Orellana M, Glineur R. Genioplasty with surgical guide using 3D-printing technology: a systematic review. J Clin Exp Dent. 2020;12(1):e85–92.
17. Shaik M, Koteswar Rao N, Kiran Kumar N, Prasanthi G. Comparison of rigid and semirigid fixation for advancement genioplasty. J Maxillofac Oral Surg. 2013;12(3):260–5.
18. Collins PC, Epker BN. Improvement in the augmentation genioplasty via suprahyoid muscle repositioning. J Maxillofac Surg. 1983;11(3):116–20.
19. Khan M, Sattar N, Erkin M. Postoperative complications in genioplasty and their association with age, gender, and type of genioplasty. Int J Dent. 2021;2021:1.

Simultaneous Bimaxillary Surgery and Rhinoplasty: Evolving Concepts in Orthofacial Surgery

12

Mirco Raffaini and Francesco Arcuri

12.1 Introduction

The nasolabial unit represents a key component of the face. The interrelation between the upper lip, teeth, maxillary alveolus and base, cheeks, and nose is important in life relationships, the perception of facial beauty, verbal and nonverbal communication, as well as in respiratory and feeding functions. The Le Fort I osteotomy is a procedure with a significant impact on midface changes, occlusion, and improvement of the smile, lip, and nose. While the procedure can positively alter the nasal septum and turbinates with functional improvements, it may have a favorable or negative impact on the shape and volume of the nose [1].

These potential negative consequences represent a critical point in orthofacial surgery. The purpose of this chapter is primarily to focus on the ways in which maxillary surgery can influence the morphology and function of the nose. Subsequently, the ways in which certain technical adjustments in the execution of the Le Fort I procedure and its repositioning can prevent negative parasitic effects will also be clarified.

We likewise will explain how the nose should be analyzed in the context of the face and profile in order to identify defects in shape, size, and airway alterations that hinder breathing. Finally, a technique will be proposed that allows simultaneous rhinoseptoplasty to refine both form and function. Of course, some mention will be made of the most current rhinoseptoplasty techniques, clarifying when the procedure can be performed simultaneously with orthognathic surgery and when it would be preferable to defer it.

12.2 Historical Perspective

The majority of maxillary deformities can be solved by three basic osteotomies: the Le Fort I-type maxillary osteotomy (LFI), the bilateral sagittal split osteotomy (BSSO) of the mandible, and the horizontal sliding osteotomy of the mandibular symphysis (genioplasty). Orthognathic surgery is frequently associated with ancillary procedures such as septoplasty, rhinoplasty, genioplasty, mandibular contouring, and facial fat grafting [2].

Recently, there has been a resurgence of global interest in preservation rhinoplasty (PR) techniques. This approach advocates for subperiosteal dissection with the preservation of nasal ligaments, limited lateral crural resection with an emphasis on suture modification techniques, and dorsal preservation through *en bloc* modification

M. Raffaini
Face Surgery, Parma, Italy

Maxillo-Facial Surgery, Milan, Italy
e-mail: mircoraffaini@facesurgery.it

F. Arcuri (✉)
IRCCS San Martino, Genoa, Italy

F. Hernández-Alfaro, A. Valls Ontañón (eds.), *Orthofacial Surgery*,
https://doi.org/10.1007/978-3-031-76185-0_12

of the dorsum while preserving the nasal keystone. Classical Joseph hump reduction techniques have long been fundamental in rhinoplasty practice and teaching. Despite variations in techniques for tissue removal (e.g., composite versus component hump reduction), osteotomies, and mid-vault reconstruction described in the literature over the decades, there is a growing critical assessment of the need for "destructive" techniques and a greater emphasis on the use of preservation techniques [3].

In the historical context, rhinoplasty trends evolve in generational epochs, often associated with revolutionary surgical techniques that demonstrate superior aesthetic or functional outcomes or a simplification of prior methodology. Landmark publications play a crucial role in these shifts. Work by John Orlando Roe in 1887 and 1891 [4], emphasizing external skin incisions and careful subcutaneous dissection, stands among the earliest publications related to modern aesthetic rhinoplasty.

In 1928 and 1929, Jacques Joseph [5] (Berlin) published monumental works focusing on reconstructive and aesthetic nasal surgery—establishing him as a pioneer in rhinoplasty. Jack Sheen's 1978 landmark text *Aesthetic Rhinoplasty* outlined surgical planning, balanced reduction and grafting, and minimizing the need for revision surgery. More recently, Dean Toriumi (Chicago) [6] published a monumental text entitled *Structure Rhinoplasty: Lessons Learned in 30 Years*, emphasizing the critical need for sound operative techniques that establish long-term structural support.

While open structural approaches advocated by these authors have become widespread, the work and techniques of innovative surgeons describing preservation concepts from the late nineteenth and early twentieth centuries were not as widely adopted. Joseph Goodale (Boston) [7] presented the idea of preserving the dorsal nasal architecture in 1899, and Oliver Lothrop [8] (Boston) described preservation techniques in 1914.

In recent times, there has been a resurgence of interest in preservation techniques, driven by theoretical functional and aesthetic benefits. Surgeons such as Gola [9] and Saban [10] (France), Tuncel [11] and Aydogdu (Turkey), Ferreira et al. [12] (Portugal), Ishida et al. [13] (Brazil), Tas [14] (Turkey), Neves et al. [15] (Portugal), and Öztürk [16] (Turkey) have contributed to the growing body of literature on preservation techniques.

In the United States, there is growing attention to the preservation ideology. Surgeons like Daniel [1] (California), along with Yves Saban [10], and Baris Cakir [17], have advocated for a fundamental change in the approach to rhinoplasty, coining the term "Preservation Rhinoplasty" (PR).

12.3 The Nasolabial Unit Concept

The intricate nasolabial region, spanning the maxilla below, features two prominent aesthetic structures: the nose and the upper lip. The Le Fort I osteotomy is commonly employed to reposition the maxilla and correct associated dentoskeletal deformities. This procedure involves the transection of perioral and perinasal musculature, accompanied by extensive periosteal degloving. A comprehensive understanding of the interconnections between the hard framework and soft tissues, particularly the muscular web, is crucial in this regard. This knowledge is essential for effectively managing the changes induced by maxillary exposure and repositioning on the nose and upper lip. Secondary alterations in the nasolabial unit following the orthognathic procedure include: (1) widening of the alar bases; (2) upturning of the nasal tip leading to increased supratip depression; (3) changes in the nasolabial angle; (4) increased prominence of the alar groove; (5) flattening, drooping, and thinning of the upper lip; (6) reduction of vermillion exposure; and (7) downturning of the commissures of the mouth. Numerous authors have proposed techniques to address these effects, often yielding variable and unpredictable or unstable outcomes. By employing appropriate surgical techniques, many undesirable secondary changes can be prevented, preserving the nose and achieving aesthetic enhancement of the lip. This approach allows for the simultaneous performance of rhinoplasty and maxillomandibular osteotomies [18].

The nasolabial unit serves as a vital aesthetic component within facial volumes and contours, reflecting intrinsic conditions related to soft-tissue distribution and thickness. Crucially, it unveils the disposition and morphology of the underlying skeletal structures. While analyzing contours is relatively straightforward due to their linear nature, we prefer to evaluate the morphology of the upper lip in its subunits in profile, namely the subnasale or angle, the lip line, and vermilion. Understanding the form of the upper lip involves considering the lower part of the nose and the subnasal inflection point. The hard support for the nasolabial unit comprises two distinct parts: the lower or dentoalveolar maxillary part and the upper or nasal part. The lower part includes the frontal teeth, their tipping, position in the maxillary alveolar structures, and the basal maxillary skeleton. The upper part in turn constitutes the lower nasal framework, characterized by a tripod resting on a strong median pedestal formed by the anterior nasal spine and the caudal third of the septum. The skin-soft tissue envelope overlies this tripod–pedestal skeleton, determining the shape of the nasal lower third and defining the subnasal position, crucial for lip tethering and curling [19].

To comprehend the nasolabial unit contour clearly and understand the supporting framework, it is essential to consider both the dentomaxillary structure and the nasal structure. The interplay between the upper and lower skeletal parts allows for addressing treatment alternately on the dentomaxillary structure, nasal structure, or both. The features of the pedestal are particularly significant in influencing the morphology of the upper lip and, indirectly, the tripod. Excessive dimensions of the pedestal, such as dorsal length, anterior projection, or caudal extension, can impact the appearance. For instance, an anteriorly enlarged pedestal may lead to a "tension nose," producing an appearance of deficient lip support. In such cases, the key lies in trimming the excessive pedestal component rather than adjusting the teeth or maxilla.

Another scenario involves excess of the caudal septum, forcing the tripod and nasal tip downward into an under-rotated or plunging tip position. Addressing the excess pedestal is essential to affect rotation in the septal caudal portion, improving both the lower nose and the nasal angle.

Various conditions, such as an overprojected and downrotated nasal tip or a deficient pedestal, may necessitate specific surgical interventions to achieve harmonious outcomes between the lower nose and the lip. Each alteration of the nasolabial unit should be studied considering both the dentomaxillary framework and the nasal cartilaginous skeleton, ensuring an integrated approach for more harmonious results in orthodontic surgical treatments.

Furthermore, the nose, being centrally positioned on the face, holds a pivotal role in the overall harmonious perception of facial features. Consequently, addressing various dentomaxillary deformities often necessitates not only a combination of orthodontics and orthognathic surgery but also a correction of nasal morphology [20].

12.4 Preoperative Evaluation of the Nose, Mandible, and Maxilla

12.4.1 Frontal View

The frontal view analysis focuses on the nasal bridge, which should form two roughly parallel lines from the brow to the tip defining points. A slight concavity is acceptable in the nasal bridge, but smooth and uninterrupted paths are expected, leading directly to an elegant, natural, and inconspicuous nasal tip. Tip defining points should be discrete, symmetrical, and appropriately spaced apart. Bulbosity to the supratip can disrupt the brow–tip lines and is detectable from the frontal view. Alar base width should be just inside the vertical lines extending from the medial canthi.

12.4.2 Lateral View

The head should be at rest in a natural position during the analysis of facial thirds, tip projection, dorsal contour, alar–columellar relation, radix, and chin position. Tip projection can be measured using various methods, and surgeons need to be aware of the potential illusion of increased tip projection due to certain maneuvers. The columella should be positioned 2–3 mm below the alar margin. The nasion, representing the deepest point of the nasofrontal angle, should be approximately 120° and align with the supratarsal crease. The maxillo-mandibular projection is evaluated considering a line perpendicular to the natural head orientation at the nasion or referring to the subnasale.

12.4.3 Basal View

In the basal view, the nose should resemble an equilateral triangle, with the upper third representing the tip lobule and the lower two-thirds corresponding to the columella. Notable features include nostril shape, columellar width, alar base, and the thickness of the alar lobules.

12.5 Operative Procedure

Traditionally, rhinoplasty was conducted at a later stage, typically 6 months or more after maxillary and mandibular osteotomies, aiming to reduce the risks associated with postoperative recovery. Challenges included intermaxillary fixation, difficulty in performing nasal-changing procedures due to midface deformation postmaxillary surgery, increased postoperative edema, and extended operating time.

However, advancements in surgical techniques, specifically the routine application of internal rigid fixation with plates and screws to the jaws, have enabled the simultaneous performance of maxillary osteotomies and rhinoplasty in a single surgical procedure. This eliminates the need for intermaxillary fixation, offering several advantages. The single surgical procedure provides improved access and visibility to structures like the septum or nasal spine during maxillary surgery. Additionally, this approach allows for a more harmonious correction of the nasolabial unit, addressing problems in a well-coordinated manner.

In the context of orthognathic surgery with a mandible-first protocol, LFI osteotomy is carried out as follows: mucosal incision on the labial side is performed between canine and canine to ensure vascular supply to the bone also via the mucosa of the maxillary fornix.

The anterior maxilla is exposed, and the nasal spine is osteotomized from the maxilla with a sharp 12 mm osteotome, leaving 1 cm of the nasal spine and the anterior nasal crest of the maxilla connected with the septum and respecting a thin sling of the lower portion of the nasolabial muscle inserted on the spine itself. After this subspinal osteotomy, the nasal mucosa is raised from the nasal floor with a periosteal elevator. The nasal septum is thus laterally pushed, luxated, and rotated by the same elevator on both sides to free it from the maxilla.

The subperiosteal dissection of the maxilla is extended to the rear through a small lateral tunnel on each side. The aim is to limit skeletal exposure to the surface strictly needed to perform osteotomy outlines. Subsequently, a low-level Le Fort I horizontal osteotomy is marked with a reciprocating saw (The OsteoPower™ System from Osteomed, Addison, TX, USA) with a 2 cm blade or, better, with an ultrasonic chisel (Mectron Medical Technology, ADC Dental, Bois d'Amont, France).

Pterygoid–maxillary disjunction is performed with a transmucosal flapless osteotomy, inserting the piezoelectric blade through a stab incision from below and laterally between the maxillary tuberosity and the pterygoid process. Then, a straight osteotome is driven through the horizontal osteotomy from the pyriform buttress back to the junction of the posterior wall of the maxillary sinus with the pterygoid plate and twisted, easily separating the pterygoid process from the maxillary tuberosity. The same procedure is repeated at the contralateral side according to the "twist technique" popularized by Hernández-Alfaro [21].

Complete mobilization of the maxilla is obtained inserting a spreader instrument in the osteotomy site at the level of the zygomatic buttress and opening it wide. All the insertions of the pterygoid muscles on the posterior maxilla are carefully detached; in the case of large advancement, the palatine neurovascular bundle is coagulated and sectioned in order to avoid stretching it with possible postoperative bleeding. Moreover, 1 cm of palatine bone is cut as well as some interfering fragment of the tuber maxilla in order to secure more freedom of the maxilla from the pterygoid plates.

After maxillary mobilization, the nasal procedures involving the nasal septum (such as inferior septal strip removal or vomer deformity), turbinates, and sinuses are easily accomplished through the oral approach, which allows for a better control of correction of the nasal airway. Care is taken to close the nasal mucosa to minimize postoperative bleeding if exposure of the inferior turbinates is clinically indicated. To set the nasal spine in its natural position avoiding septal distortion, it is imperative to prepare adequate room in the upper anterior maxilla with a bur, according to the tongue-in-groove principle. Osteotomy gaps are filled using a homologous bone graft block tailored to the defects. Intubation is converted into orotracheal intubation, with the tube positioned in the center of the lower lip to allow for the PR procedure.

After a standard open approach, subperichondral and subperiosteal dissection is extended to the radix of the nose and the nasal bones. After complete dissection, a bilateral transverse nasal osteotomy and intraoral lateral nasal osteotomies are performed. Then, the cartilaginous septum is exposed through the anterior access; the perpendicular plate of the ethmoid is osteotomized at the level of the superficial strip of quadrangular cartilage removed to entirely mobilize the nasal pyramid. In the case of a "let-down procedure," an internal lateral nasal osteotomy is implemented by transoral bilateral osseous wedge resection from the frontal ascending processes of the maxillary bones, using a piezoelectric device. The septum T is lowered and stabilized with two to three stitches at the underlying residual septum (side-to-side or hedge-to-hedge, depending on the existence of septal deviation). Finally, after modification of the osseous and cartilaginous nasal vault, tip-plasty is addressed according to the preservation principles, depending on the need for reduction, reshaping, rotation, and projection of the tip.

Subtypes of dorsal preservation (DP) are reported according to a recent classification: type I (full let down), type II (bone scoring + full let down), type III (bone ostectomy + basal osteotomies + cartilage let down), type IV (bone scoring + cartilage let down), and type V (bone scoring + upper cartilage rim resection) [22–24].

Type I is characterized by osteotomy of the radix and lateral ostectomy (Figs. 12.1 and 12.2); it is performed in patients where both the bony and cartilaginous dorsum are relatively flat and aesthetically acceptable. In the case of full let down and bone scoring, DP is classified as type II (Figs. 12.3 and 12.4). Type III is a "hybrid technique" characterized by standard resection to the bony dorsum and closure of the open bony roof with classical osteotomies. It is indicated in patients with an unpleasant bony dorsum or excessive convexity. Type IV is known as cartilage-only DP; in this technique, the dorsal cartilage is preserved and lowered, and progressive resection of the bony roof is performed until it is as thin as a membranous bony cap which remains above the upper lateral cartilage. It is indicated in patients with short nasal bones and a large cartilaginous component of the dorsum. Finally, type V is characterized by bone scoring and upper cartilage rim resection; it is indicated in patients where small and slight modifications of the bony and cartilaginous back are necessary.

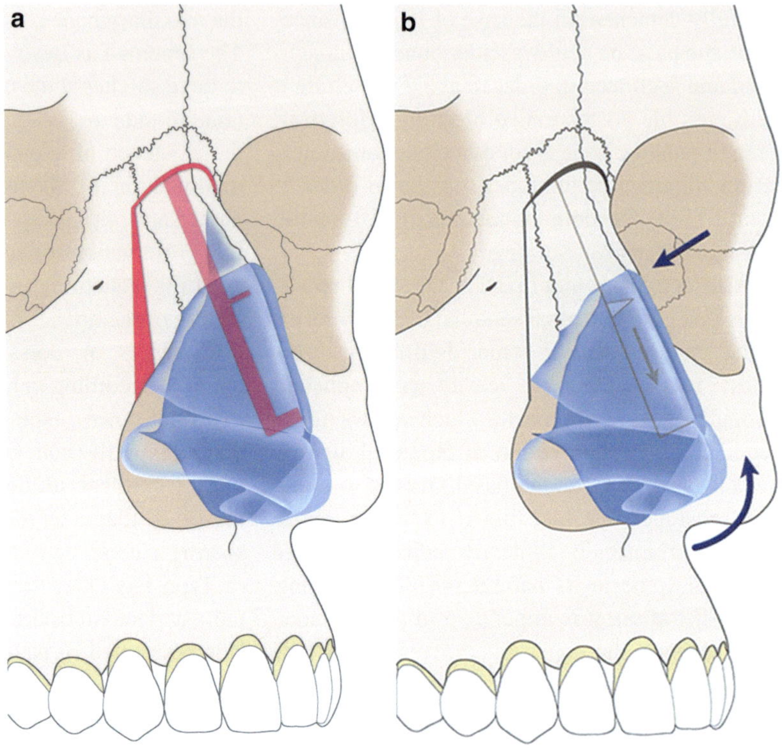

Fig. 12.1 (**a** and **b**) Type 1 dorsal preservation

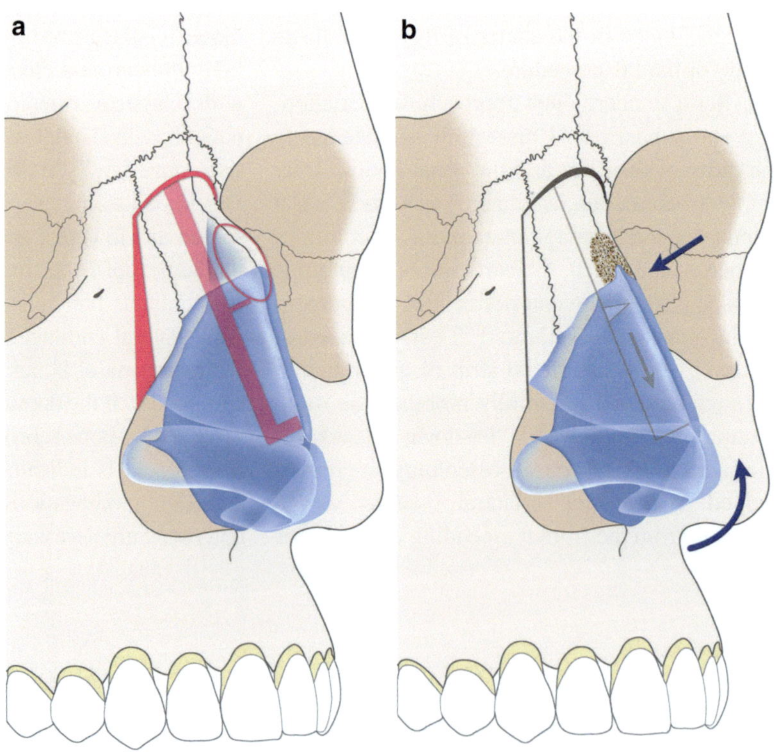

Fig. 12.2 (**a** and **b**) Preoperative and postoperative clinical views of simultaneous bimaxillary surgery (counterclockwise rotation) plus genioplasty and type 1 dorsal preservation

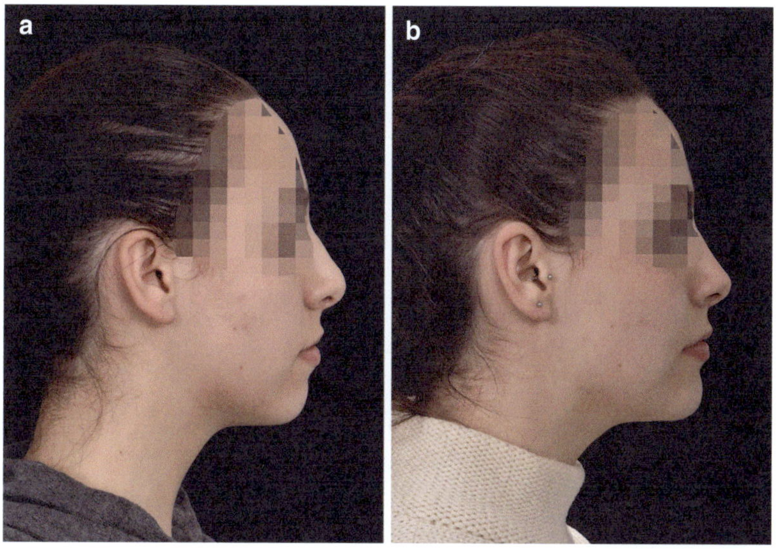

Fig. 12.3 (**a** and **b**) Type 2 dorsal preservation

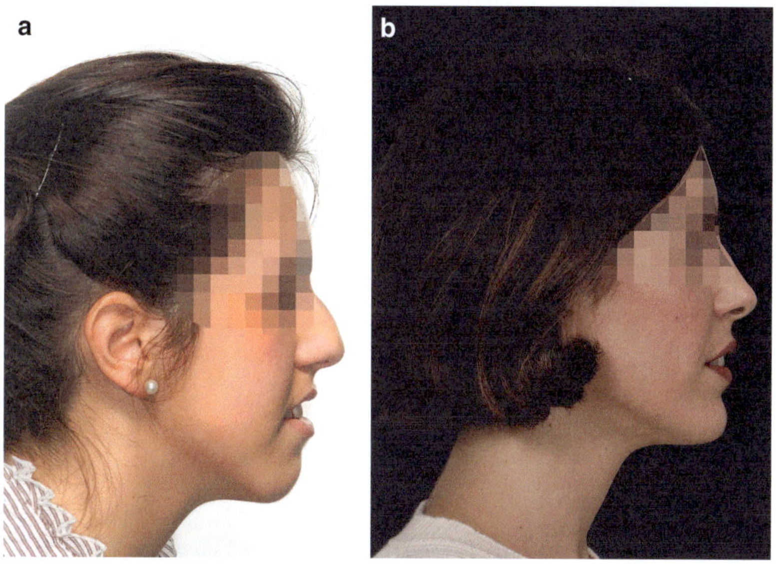

Fig. 12.4 (**a** and **b**) Preoperative and postoperative clinical views of simultaneous bimaxillary surgery (counterclockwise rotation) plus genioplasty and type 2 dorsal preservation

12.6 Key Points

Authors have proposed various soft-tissue repositioning and closure techniques to control these changes, but predictability and stable success have not been consistently achieved. To address these concerns, some authors have suggested modifying the osteotomy outline, cutting beneath the nasal spine to preserve the integrity of the nasolabial muscle. This technique involves a small mucosal incision and limited periosteal dissection, working in two lateral tunnels and performing osteotomies at a lower level in respect of the teeth apexes. The goal is a more conservative approach to soft-tissue structures. This modified approach has shown success in minimizing the adverse effects of Le Fort I osteotomy on the nose and upper lip. Additionally, in cases of pre-existing nasal alterations, a simultaneous rhinoplasty can be performed after the orthognathic procedure. The usual sequence involves the orthognathic procedure as the initial step, followed by rhinoplasty after converting intubation to allow the required access.

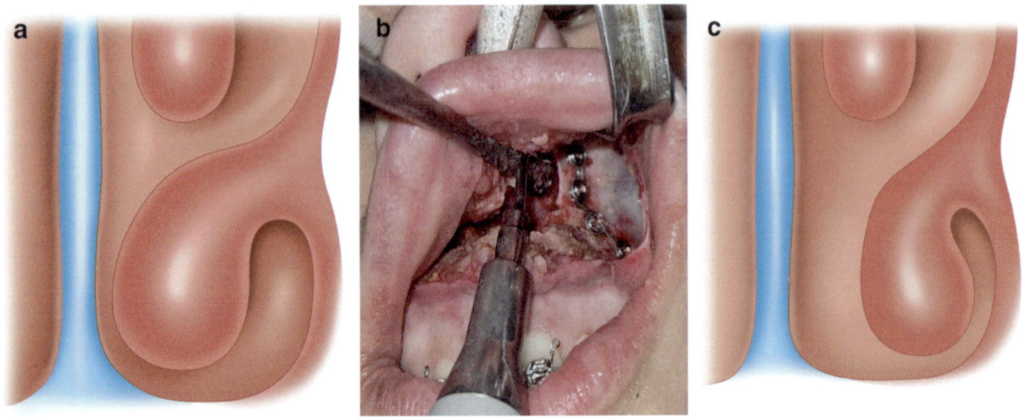

Fig. 12.5 (**a–c**) Ostectomy of the inferior turbinate in order to lateralize it

The let-down operation is based on three operative concepts: (1) preservation of the soft-tissue nasal envelope by dissecting in a subperichondral–subperiosteal plane with the preservation of the fibrous nasal ligaments; (2) preservation of the osteocartilaginous (or only cartilaginous) dorsum by maintaining the integrity of the middle third and removing a strip of cartilage from the septum to lower the bridge; and (3) preservation of the alar cartilages with tensioning and suturing techniques limiting excisional procedures or grafting [25–29].

The advantages of the piezoelectric device are as follows: (1) lateralization of the turbinates is not based on a greenstick fracture but on a piezo-assisted cut, which prevents recurrence; the incision for access of the insert is limited and prevents bleeding; (2) precise removal of a posterior strip of bone septum; and (3) lateral ostectomy and osteotomy of the radix of the nose (Figs. 12.5 and 12.6).

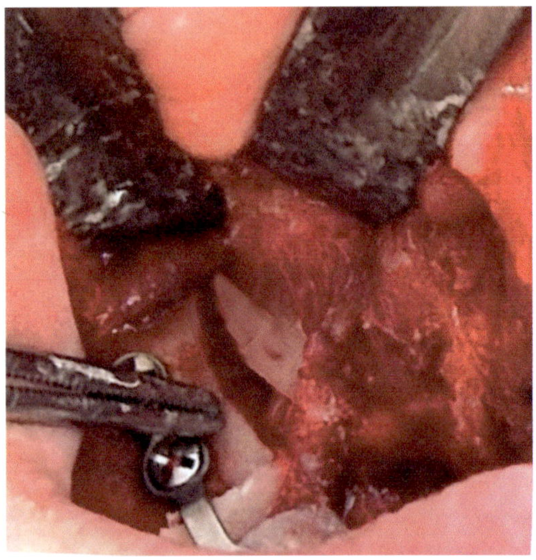

Fig. 12.6 Intraoperative detail of the transoral osteotomy of the nasal wall

Several authors have analyzed the concerns of patients seeking secondary rhinoplasty both for structural rhinoplasty and PR. Regarding structural rhinoplasty, in a retrospective study of 100 secondary rhinoplasties, Constantian [30] found that the most common reasons for redone surgery were correction of a new deformity and failure to correct the original deformity. Nassab [31] in turn conducted a retrospective review of 109 cases in which septal deviation accounted for 32.1% as a cause of revision. Hellings [32] found that 15% of the patients presented functional problems and 30% presented a combination of aesthetic and functional concerns ($n = 43$). Lee et al. [33], in a study of 100 revision rhinoplasties, found that 65% of the patients presented some airway occlusion, and septal deviation accounted for 29%, with an incidence of secondary rhinoplasty of 5–15%. Yu [34] et al. in turn reported an incidence of airway occlusion of 61%, while Foda [35] reported an incidence of airway occlusion of 68%.

12.7 Discussion

The advantages of PR [10–17, 21–29] when compared to conventional structural rhinoplasty are as follows: (1) preservation of the keystone area and attachment of the upper lateral cartilages to the septum; (2) maintenance of dorsal aesthetic lines; (3) preservation of the internal nasal valve; (4) greater precision in correcting the deviation of the nasal pyramid in the coronal plane; and (5) a lesser need for revision. However, patients with a large bony component, deep nasofrontal angle, or irregular bony pyramid are not ideal candidates for PR.

Various techniques can be employed to reduce and reposition septal cartilage before osteocartilaginous pyramid mobilization. They can be grouped into the following categories: (1) high-septal strip/subdorsal resection (Saban's modified Cottle high subdorsal resection [10]) in the case of a dorsal hump <4 mm with a high septal deviation; (2) mid-septal strip/subdorsal flaps in the case of a slight crooked nose (Ishida's septal strip excision closer to the mid-aspect of the septum [13], Ferreira's technique [12]); (3) low-septal strip if there is a disease condition along the connection of the anterior nasal spine and maxillary crest (Cottle [4] or Finocchi's [36] "SPQR" simplified preservation quick rhinoplasty); and (4) bony dorsal preservation in the case of a crooked nose with straight dorsal aesthetic lines, where there is no disease condition at the septal base [16, 17].

The advantages of the combined technique with a transoral approach to the inner part of the nasal cavity made possible by orthognathic surgery are as follows: (1) superior visibility during ostectomy of the inferior turbinate in order to lateralize it; (2) transoral precise basal ostectomy/osteotomy, avoiding undermining of the lateral nasal walls; (3) effective management of high septal deviations of the bony components (perpendicular plate of the ethmoid and vomer bone); (4) the possibility of fixing the nasal spine (attached to the cartilaginous septum) in the center of the upper jaw; and (5) the possibility of reconstructing the nasolabial muscles in order to control the width of the nostrils.

The disadvantages of the combined approach in turn are as follows: (1) difficulty in predicting the nasal tip position after LFI; (2) a longer surgery time; and (3) difficulty changing the tube if the airway is not clearly visualized. Although Pary [37] described submental intubation for combined cases, we do not consider it effective in this context due to the difficulty in mobilizing the mandible. We reserve it for complex traumatology cases.

The indications of staged rhinoplasty are (1) cleft nose and syndromic patients; (2) secondary rhinoplasty (need for nasal reconstruction); (3) a post-traumatic severely altered nose; (4) complex facial asymmetries; (5) consistent downgrafting maxillary repositioning; and (6) great mandibular advancement (>15 mm).

It is important to mention that deformities of various aspects of the nose, such as the dorsum, nasal length, septal deviation, nasal tip width, and asymmetries, tend to remain relatively unchanged following orthognathic surgery. Consequently, these deformities require targeted surgical corrections. In contrast, aspects related to the position of the nasal tip, including rotation, projection, and nasolabial changes, are influenced by bimaxillary surgery and warrant accurate prediction and planning.

In a study led by Waite [38], it was found that 94% of 22 patients who underwent combined orthognathic surgery and rhinoplasty expressed satisfaction with the final results of orthognathic surgery, while 84% were content with the outcomes of rhinoplasty. Berlin et al. [39] examined outcomes of orthognathic surgery alone and in conjunction with supplementary procedures (such as septoplasty, rhinoplasty, and genioplasty) in the United States between 1999 and 2011. They identified an overall complication rate of 5.4% in the analyzed group, with higher rates among pediatric patients (under 18 years of age).

Another recent article by Sun and Steinbacher [40] further supports the idea of performing rhinoplasty and orthognathic surgery simultaneously. In their study involving 12 patients, no revision procedures were needed during the 18-month follow-up period, and the patients reported high levels of satisfaction with both the functional and aesthetic outcomes.

References

1. Daniel RK. The preservation rhinoplasty: a new rhinoplasty revolution. Aesthet Surg J. 2018;38(02):228–9.
2. Posnick JC, Agnihotri N. Consequences and management of nasal airway obstruction in the dentofacial deformity patient. Curr Opin Otolaryngol Head Neck Surg. 2010;18(4):323–31.
3. Azizzadeh B, Reilly M. Dorsal hump reduction and osteotomies. Clin Plast Surg. 2016;43(01):47–58.
4. Cottle MH. John Orlando Roe, pioneer in modern rhinoplasty. Arch Otolaryngol. 1964;80:22–7.
5. Bhattacharya S. Jacques Joseph: father of modern aesthetic surgery. Indian J Plast Surg. 2008;41:S3–8.
6. Toriumi D. Structure rhinoplasty: lessons learned in 30 years. Chicago: DMT Publishers; 2018.
7. Goodale JL. A new method for the operative correction of exaggerated roman nose. Boston Med Surg J. 1899;140:112.
8. Lothrop OA. An operation for correcting the aquiline nasal deformity: the use of a new instrument. Report of a case. Boston Med Surg J. 1914;170(22):835–7.
9. Gola R. Functional and esthetic rhinoplasty. Aesth Plast Surg. 2003;27(05):390–6.
10. Saban Y, Braccini F, Polselli R. [Rhinoplasty: morphodynamic anatomy of rhinoplasty. Interest of conservative rhinoplasty]. Rev Laryngol Otol Rhinol (Bord). 2006;127(1–2):15–22.
11. Tuncel U, Aydogdu O. The probable reasons for dorsal hump problems following let-down/push-down rhinoplasty and solution proposals. Plast Reconstr Surg. 2019;144(03):378e–85e.
12. Ferreira MG, Monteiro D, Reis C, Almeida e Sousa C. Spare roof technique: a middle third new technique. Facial Plast Surg. 2016;32(01):111–6.
13. Ishida J, Ishida LC, Ishida LH, Vieira JC, Ferreira MC. Treatment of the nasal hump with preservation of the cartilaginous framework. Plast Reconstr Surg. 1999;103(06):1729–33, discussion 1734–5.
14. Taş S. Dorsal roof technique for dorsum preservation in rhinoplasty. Aesthet Surg J. 2020;40(03):263–75.
15. Neves JC, Arancibia Tagle D, Dewes W, Larrabee W. The split preservation rhinoplasty: "the Vitruvian Man split maneuver". Eur J Plast Surg. 2020;43:323–33.
16. Öztürk G. Push-down technique without osteotomy: a new approach. Aesth Plast Surg. 2020;44(03):891–901.
17. Cakir B, Dogan T, Oreroglu AR, Daniel RK. Rhinoplasty: surface aesthetics and surgical techniques. Aesthet Surg J. 2013;33(3):363–75.
18. Raffaini M, Cocconi R, Spinelli G, Agostini T. Simultaneous rhinoseptoplasty and orthognathic surgery: outcome analysis of 250 consecutive patients using a modified Le Fort I osteotomy. Aesth Plast Surg. 2018;42(4):1090–100.
19. Marion F, Mercier JM, Odri GA, Perrin JP, Longis J, Kün-Darbois JD, Corre P, Bertin H. Associated relaps factors in Le Fort I osteotomy. A retrospective study of 54 cases. J Stomatol Oral Maxillofac Surg. 2019;120(5):419–27.
20. Arnett GW, Gunson MJ. Facial planning for orthodontists and oral surgeons. Am J Orthod Dentofacial Orthop. 2004;126(290):33.
21. Hernández-Alfaro F, Guijarro-Martínez R. "Twist technique" for pterygomaxillary dysjunction in minimally invasive Le Fort I osteotomy. J Oral Maxillofac Surg. 2013;71(2):389–92.
22. Gonçalves Ferreira M, Toriumi DM. A practical classification system for dorsal preservation rhinoplasty techniques. Facial Plast Surg Aesthet Med. 2021;23(3):153–5.
23. Robotti E, Chauke-Malinga NY, Leone F. A modified dorsal split preservation technique for nasal humps with minor bony component: a preliminary report. Aesthetic Plast Surg. 2019;43(5):1257–68.
24. Kosins AM, Daniel RK. Decision making in preservation rhinoplasty: a 100 case series with one-year follow-up. Aesthet Surg J. 2020;40(1):34–48.
25. Drumheller GH. Septal reconstruction in the deficient nose. Rhinology. 1976;14(4):189–92. PMID: 794982.
26. Hall JA, Peters MD, Hilger PA. Modification of the Skoog dorsal reduction for preservation of the middle nasal vault. Arch Facial Plast Surg. 2004;6(2):105–10.
27. Skoog T. A method of hump reduction in rhinoplasty: a technique for preservation of the nasal roof. Arch Otolaryngol. 1966;83:283–7.
28. Sabeti F, Tehrani AN. A new technique for reconstruction of the nasal dorsum: underlay autografting. Arch Facial Plast Surg. 2002;4:141–8.
29. Cerkes N. Concurrent elevation of the upper lateral cartilage perichondrium and nasal bone periosteum for management of dorsum: the perichondro-periosteal flap. Aesthet Surg J. 2013;33(6):899–914.
30. Constantian MB. Differing characteristics in 100 consecutive secondary rhinoplasty patients following closed versus open surgical approaches. Plast Reconstr Surg. 2002;109(6):2097–111.
31. Nassab R, Matti B. Presenting concerns and surgical management of secondary rhinoplasty. Aesthet Surg J. 2015;35(2):137–44.
32. Hellings PW, Nolst Trenité GJ. Long-term patient satisfaction after revision rhinoplasty. Laryngoscope. 2007;117(6):985–9.
33. Lee M, Zwiebel S, Guyuron B. Frequency of the preoperative flaws and commonly required maneuvers to correct them: a guide to reducing the revision rhinoplasty rate. Plast Reconstr Surg. 2013;132(4):769–76.
34. Yu K, Kim A, Pearlman SJ. Functional and aesthetic concerns of patients seeking revision rhinoplasty. Arch Facial Plast Surg. 2010;12:291–7.

35. Foda HM. Rhinoplasty for the multiply revised nose. Am J Otolaryngol. 2005;26:28–34.
36. Finnochi V. SPQR technique. Personal communication, preservation rhinoplasty meeting, Rome, Italy; 2019.
37. Pary A. Rhinoplasty in oral and maxillofacial surgery. Personal communication, COBRAC: Congreso Brasileiro de Chirugia e Traumatologia Bucomaxilofacial, Florianopolis, Brasil; 2022.
38. Waite PD, Matukas VJ, Sarver DM. Simultaneous rhinoplasty procedures in orthognathic surgery. Int J Oral Maxillofac Surg. 1988;17:298.
39. Berlin NL, Tuggle CT, Steinbacher DM. Improved short term outcomes following orthognathic surgery are associated with high-volume centers. Plast Reconstr Surg. 2016;138(2):273e–81e.
40. Sun AH, Steinbacher DM. Orthognathic surgery and rhinoplasty: simultaneous or staged? Plast Reconstr Surg. 2018;141:322.

13 Ancillary Procedures in Orthofacial Surgery: Malarplasty, Lipofilling, Bichectomy, and Jaw Angles

Tulsi Roy and Derek M. Steinbacher

13.1 Introduction

Beyond functional concerns, orthognathic surgery can transform the facial profile and impart a rejuvenated and youthful façade. By contrast, a hypoplastic or underdeveloped skeletal framework can exacerbate an aged or sullen appearance. Orthognathic strategies to address these concerns are aimed at expanding the craniofacial skeleton to counteract skeletal disproportion and improve the height and projection of the middle and lower thirds of the face [1]. By restoring structural harmony, the facial profile can be optimized, the soft tissue envelope resuspended, and tension on ligamentous facial support reset. While orthognathic intervention alone can yield dramatic functional changes, adjunctive procedures such as facial implants, fat grafting or fillers, liposuction, and skin tightening can provide aesthetically optimal results. This chapter will focus on several ancillary aesthetic interventions, their indications, and relative advantages and drawbacks.

T. Roy (✉) · D. M. Steinbacher
Section of Plastic and Reconstructive Surgery, Yale University School of Medicine,
New Haven, CT, USA
e-mail: tulsi.roy@yale.edu; derek.steinbacher@yale.edu

13.2 Facial Implants: Malarplasty and Angle Augmentation

Alloplastic facial augmentation is especially useful to highlight the malar eminence, mandibular angle, and chin, and it can be performed alone or in conjunction with orthognathic surgery or staged rhinoplasty [2]. While the use of soft tissue fillers and fat grafting has been increasingly popularized owing to their convenience and ease of use, there is a limit to which soft-tissue augmentation can compensate for an overall deficient skeletal framework. Skeletal augmentation serves as an important tool for the aesthetic and orthognathic surgeon to enhance facial contours and convexities with a high degree of stability and reliability.

The ideal implant material is one that is biocompatible, customizable, resistant to migration or extrusion, and easily removed if necessary. Resistance to infection is beneficial, as many facial implants are placed through intraoral incisions and may be susceptible to bacterial contamination with oral flora. If extraoral incisions are planned, additional attention should be given to implant malleability in order to limit the incision length for larger devices. Implant material ranges from titanium, silicone, high-density polyethylene (Medpor), polyamide mesh (Supramid), Teflon, porous polytetrafluoroethylene carbon, to Gore-Tex [3]. Each of these materials has its advantages and disadvantages:

F. Hernández-Alfaro, A. Valls Ontañón (eds.), *Orthofacial Surgery*,
https://doi.org/10.1007/978-3-031-76185-0_13

Titanium implants, though necessitate custom fabrication, are strong, lightweight, and osseointegrate well without the risk of bone resorption or capsular contracture. Particularly in the chin, silicone rubber is frequently favored by many for its decreased cost, lower infection risk, malleability, ease of intraoperative contouring, and capsule formation that facilitates straightforward future explantation. Porous devices, such as Medpor implants, are preferred by some surgeons and have a decreased risk of implant migration compared to silicone due to their propensity for fibrous tissue ingrowth.

Complications of alloplastic augmentation include infection, extrusion, malposition, implant migration, capsular contracture, nerve injury, and bone resorption. The risk of implant infection is low but is cited as high as 5–7% in the literature [4]. This is typically from implant contamination with oral or skin flora in the early postoperative period, though late abscess formation can occur from contamination and bacterial seeding from more distant infection [5]. For this reason, implant placement in patients with active infection, significant periodontal disease, or poorly controlled diabetes should be avoided. While most implant infection can be salvaged with early administration of antibiotics, this endeavor is more challenging for porous implants that are more likely to remain chronically contaminated. Immediate explantation and antibiotics are recommended in the setting of fistula formation and implant extrusion. The decision to proceed with reaugmentation should only be considered after infection has completely resolved. A history of infection of nonporous devices can predispose patients to future capsular contracture, in which overexuberant capsule formation results in palpable or visible deformation of the overlying soft tissue [6]. This is more likely in cases of supraperiosteal pocket creation or patients with very thin skin envelopes [4].

Overdissection of an implant pocket or inadequate implant fixation may lead to implant malposition. Bone resorption can also occur from the direct pressure of an implant or micromotion within its pocket, but this is usually not of significant functional or aesthetic consequence unless the device overlies sensitive structures like tooth roots. Finally, infraorbital or mental nerve injury during pocket dissection and implant placement can occur. Regional numbness is a common postoperative complaint in patients undergoing malar, chin, or angle implant placement due to neuropraxia from dissection and retraction, rather than direct nerve transection [7]. Persistent compression of the nerve from the arms of an implant should be considered if no improvement in paresthesia is noted after several weeks [4]. In these instances, the implant should be removed, and the whole implant should be either repositioned or trimmed to accommodate the nerve [8].

Computer-aided design and manufacturing has changed the field of both orthognathic surgery and facial skeletal augmentation This involves the manufacture of dimensionally accurate physical models of human anatomy derived from medical image data [9]. While stock silicone or Medpor implants do exist and are used with relative frequency, three-dimensional planning and custom fabrication allow for evaluation and correction of more sophisticated anatomic deficiencies. Furthermore, the use of custom devices results in decreased time spent in the aesthetic guesswork of intraoperatively modifying or contouring implants, obviating the need for sizers. In patients with asymmetry, mirroring the contralateral side to duplicate its contour with a high degree of precision permits very reliable skeletal restoration and augmentation. The drawbacks to virtual surgical planning include initial upfront cost and time of scans, fabrication, and coordination, though a large percentage of this cost is recouped in decreased operative time [10].

13.2.1 Malar Implants

Malar fullness is associated with a youthful and healthy appearance. By contrast, malar deficiency can impart a gaunt or aged look, which can be accompanied by poor soft tissue support and scleral show. Malar flattening can occur from a variety of factors: normal age-related bone resorption and soft tissue deflation, a history of facial trauma, or congenital deficiency that frequently occurs in concert with overall maxillary retrusion. The malar area should be assessed on frontal and lateral views, with the projection of the zygomatic arch representing the widest point of convexity between the infratemporal region and the tragus [11]. On the lateral profile, an aesthetic malar contour is represented by a gentle curve starting anterior to the ear and extending along the anterior cheek mass. Its position relative to the anterior corneal plane, a vertical plumb line drawn from the most projected aspect of the globe, can determine the adequacy of malar projection and define a positive or negative vector [12].

While soft tissue filler or autologous fat injection can be used to disguise malar skeletal deficiency, patients with significant negative vectors, deflation, and scleral show will most likely benefit from malar implants, which can also be coupled with simultaneous soft-tissue augmentation for a more anatomic reconstruction. Malar implants can be placed transorally, transconjunctivally, or transcutaneously via subciliary or rhytidectomy incisions [11]. The approach used is largely based on surgeon comfort and type of concomitant procedures. Should periorbital or transcutaneous approaches be utilized, a more malleable implant material should be considered to limit the incision size, and judicious pocket dissection should be undertaken to maintain the implant position. In our experience, the intraoral approach through an upper vestibular incision provides optimal exposure of the malar region and infraorbital nerve, obviating the need for an external scar [2]. After incising the oral mucosa, a subperiosteal dissection can be carried out to expose the zygomatic body, arch, and infraorbital nerve. We favor the use of precontoured custom titanium implants to decrease the risk of asymmetry and implant malposition. We secure these devices with at least two monocortical screws to prevent implant migration (Fig. 13.1). When presented with a unilateral deformity from trauma, the contralateral malar eminence and zygomatic arch are mirrored to create a prefabricated implant for symmetry. Finally, we use autologous fat injection to provide additional soft tissue bulk and mitigate implant palpability. Of note, we frequently perform malar augmentation at the time of index orthognathic surgery, given the exposure already provided by the Le Fort 1 osteotomy. When planning implants for this setting, care should be taken to design the implant with consideration to the area of available bone stock remaining for maxillary fixation.

13.2.2 Jaw Angle Implants

The jawline and, more specifically, the mandibular angle have been appreciated as part of a youthful, well-supported face for both men and women. Outside of significant angle asymmetry, many patients may not recognize these specific aesthetic concerns even with moderate deficiencies. With the increasing popularity of male plastic surgery, however, angle augmentation is becoming better recognized in providing a stronger, squarer, more masculine jawline. A reduced ramal height and width, by contrast, imparts a softer, more ovoid and feminine facial appearance [13]. Physical examination of a patient with a deficient jaw angle may yield hollowing in the region or a high mandibular plane angle. Patients with retrognathia, shortened rami-condylar units, or TMJ resorption are more likely to have a high mandibular plane angle, a finding that should also be obvious on lateral cephalometric radiographs or computed tomography scans [2, 14].

Compared to the chin, the jaw angle is a less well-defined structure, and no precise cephalometric measurements exist to delineate its relationship with the rest of the craniofacial skeleton. That said, a favorable mandibular angle is one that maintains good ramus length below the ear and possesses an angle less than 105 degrees. The bigonial width should ideally be equivalent to the bitemporal width and approximate or be slightly less than bizygomatic width for a masculine or feminine appearance, respectively [14]. Interventions to augment the mandibular angle with standard commercially available implants preferentially address its vertical length or lateral width, though significant asymmetries or altered anatomy from previous surgery or trauma may warrant the use of custom-designed implants to

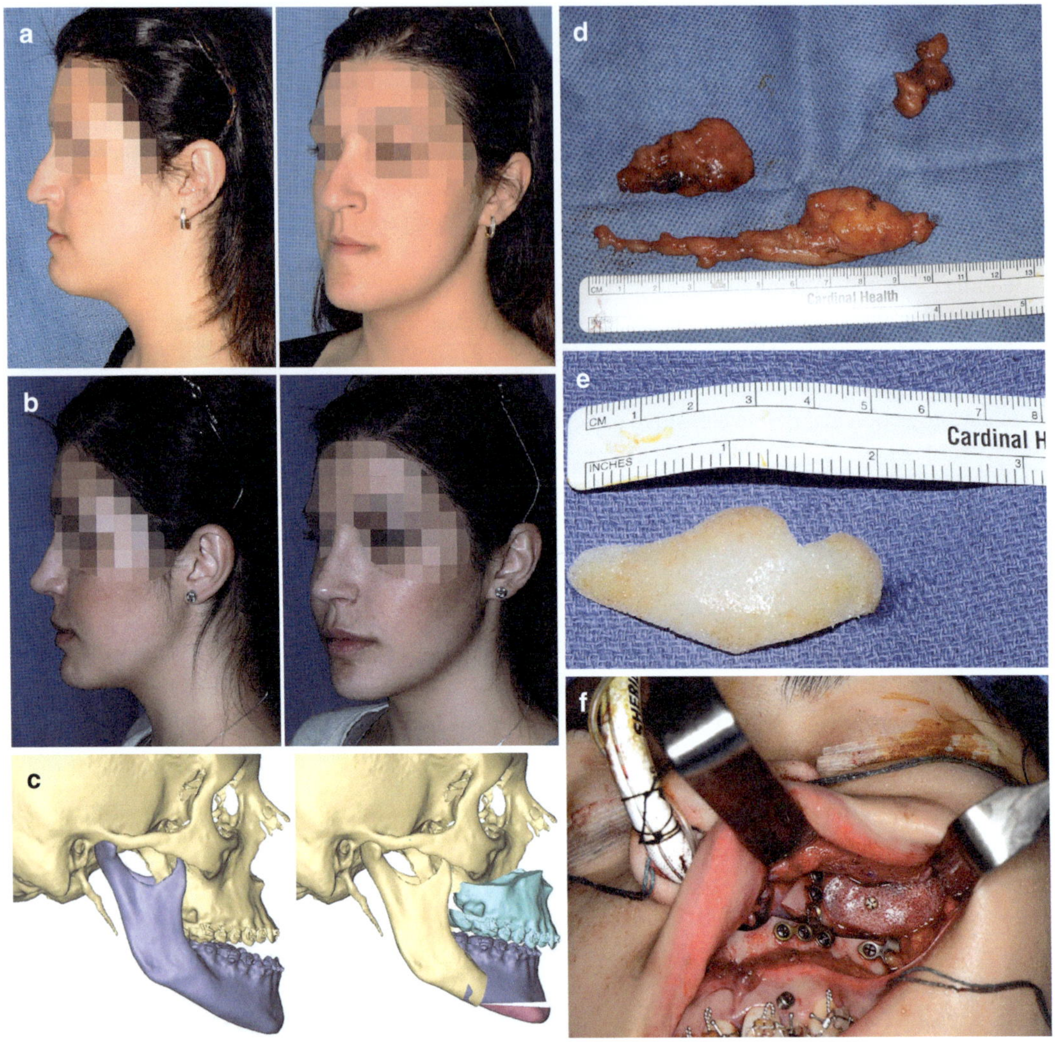

Fig. 13.1 Malar implants and buccal fat pad excision. (**a**) Preoperative and (**b**) postoperative frontal and profile photographs of a patient with improved malar projection and sculpted appearance after orthognathic surgery, bilateral malar implant placement, buccal fat excision, and staged septorhinoplasty. (**c**) Virtual simulated plan demonstrating osteotomies and orthognathic movements to address class III malocclusion, anterior open bite, and vertical microgenia. (**d**) Photo of resected buccal fat. (**e**) Medpor malar implant. (**f**) In-situ placement of the left Medpor malar implant. Note the placement and design of the implant with consideration to orthognathic maxillary plates as well as screw fixation

achieve symmetry and aesthetic balance [9]. Implant selection and goals of reconstruction should be made with the consideration of mandibular plane angle and facial balance visible from the frontal view. Patients with a steep mandibular plane angle have inadequate ramus length, so if stock implants are to be considered, vertical lengthening should be favored (Fig. 13.2). Most men with a normal mandibular plane angle typically lack bigonial width rather than ramus height, so lateral widening style implants are good choices for most male patients [14].

The surgical approach to the angle is typically intraorally through posterior vestibular incisions, though transcutaneous approaches have been described. Should angle implant placement be

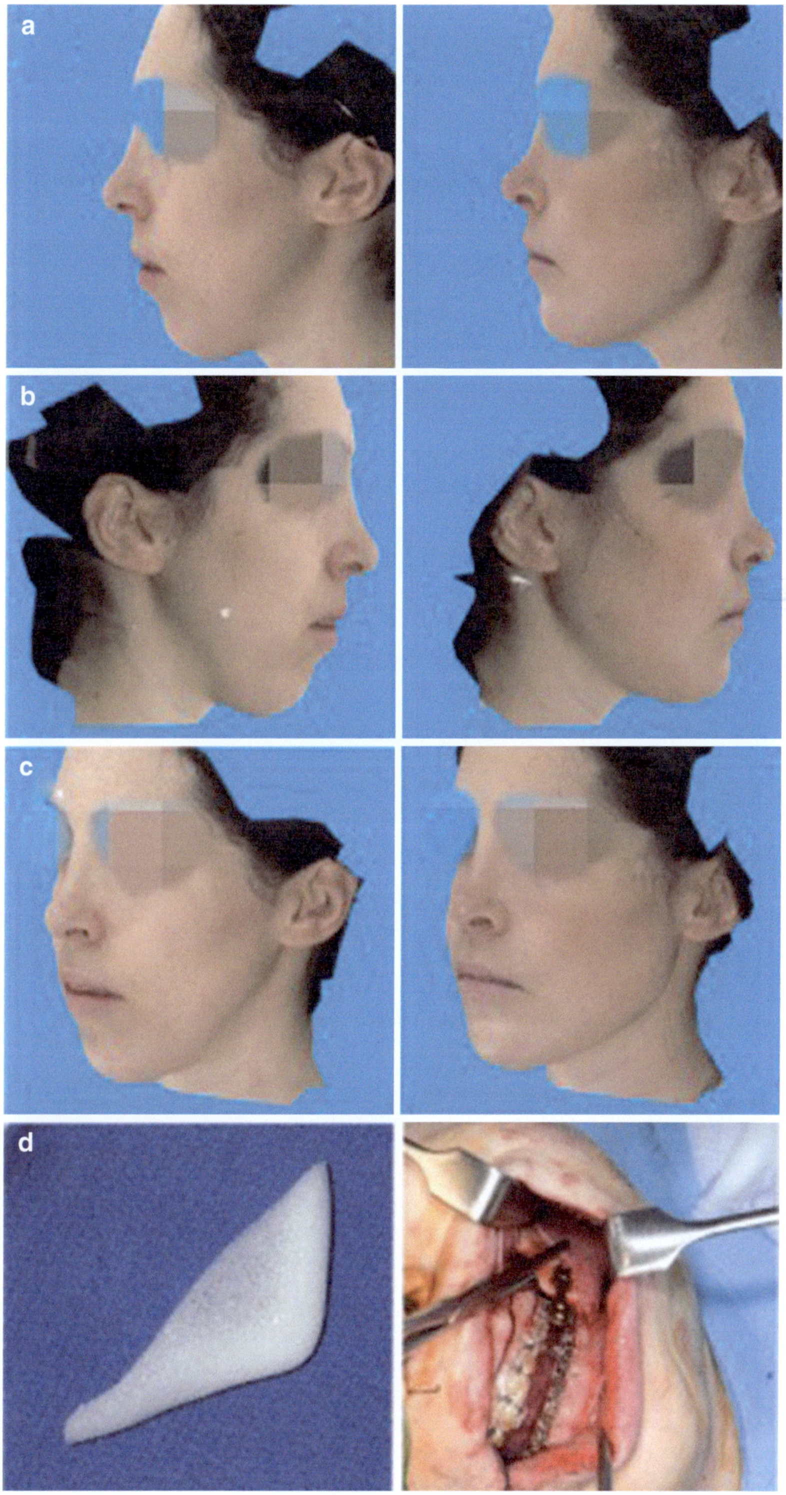

Fig. 13.2 Medpor jaw angle implants. (**a**–**c**) Preoperative (left) and postoperative (right) photographs of a patient with malocclusion, high occlusal plane angle, and deficiency and hollowing at bilateral jaw angles. (**d**) Left Medpor angle implant on the surgical field (left) and in situ (right). Note the positioning and placement of the implant prior to BSSO fixation

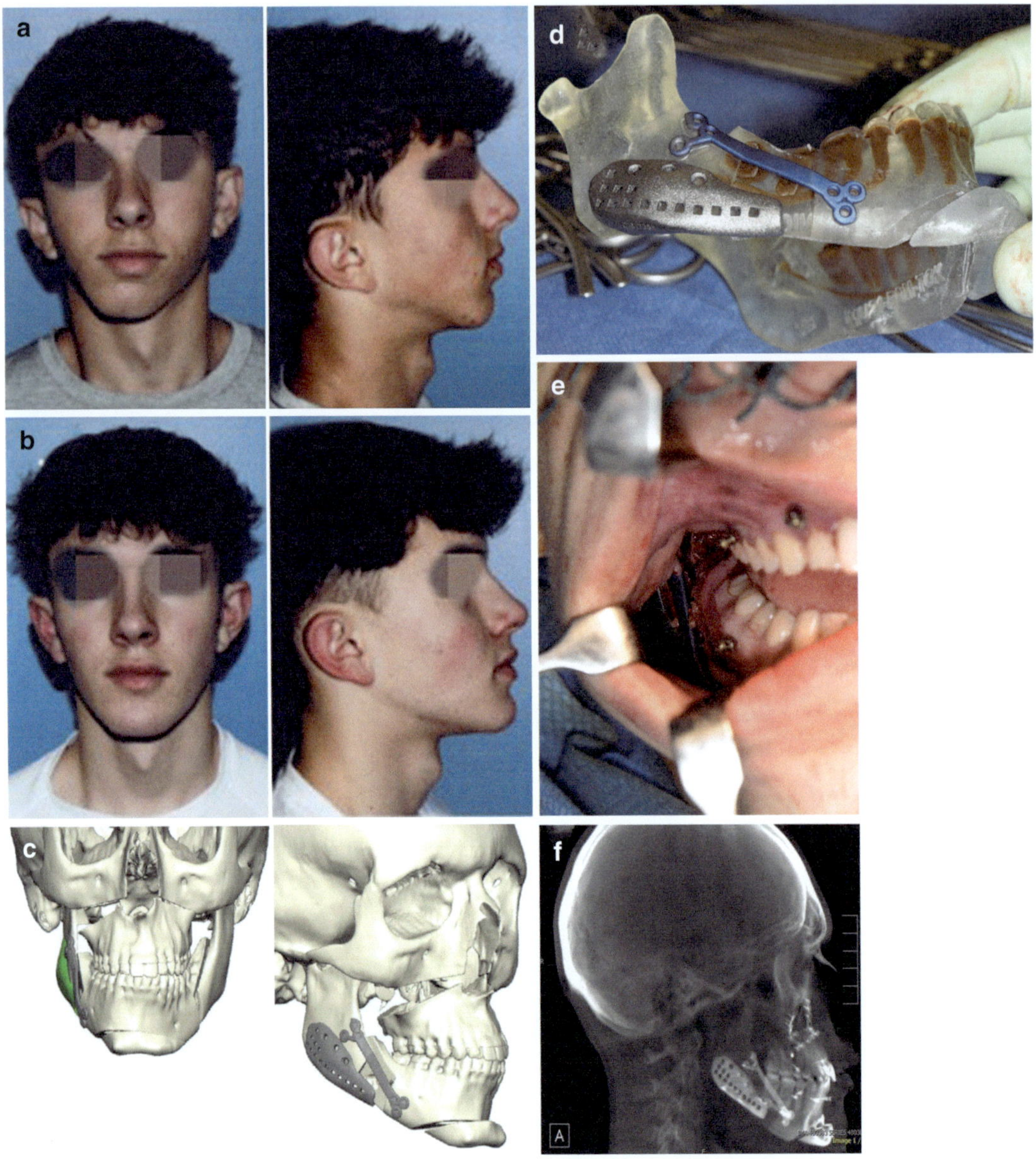

Fig. 13.3 Titanium jaw angle implants. (**a**) Preoperative photographs of a patient with facial asymmetry, chin deviation, and deficient right mandibular angle (**b**) Postoperative images showing improvement in facial balance and symmetry following orthognathic surgery and right mandibular angle implant placement. (**c**) Virtual surgical plan demonstrating orthognathic osteotomies with 3D-printed titanium right angle implant in addition to custom BSSO plate. Green represents the mirrored contralateral normal jaw angle. (**d**) Anticipated right mandibular angle implant and custom BSSO plate on a stereolithic model. Note the design of the implant with consideration to orthognathic hardware. (**e**) In situ photograph of right 3D-printed custom titanium angle implant during surgery. (**f**) Lateral cephalogram demonstrating right angle implant and orthognathic surgical hardware

combined with orthognathic surgery, the typical incision used for bilateral sagittal split osteotomy can be used (Fig. 13.3). Once the external oblique ridge is exposed, lateral subperiosteal dissection can be carried out to the posterior mandibular border. Inferior and posterior dissection is key to avoiding implant malposition, so the use of a J-stripper or curved periosteal elevator may be useful to provide adequate exposure while maintaining the integrity of the pterygomasseteric sling and avoiding neurovascular structures and the retromandibular vein [2]. Should the pterygomasseteric sling be partially or totally disinserted, masseter retraction will yield an unaesthetic high muscle bulge when chewing and unfavorable visibility or skeletonization of the implant [15]. Implant positioning is challenging in this region, as the posterior border of the implant is difficult to visualize in the deep recesses of the pocket. The use of custom implants can aid in positioning as their pre-contoured undersurface makes them more likely to "lock into place." As the mandibular border is a mobile surface, intraoral or transcutaneous implant fixation with screws is critical to prevent implant malposition and migration.

13.3 Fat Grafting

Autologous fat grafting can restore atrophied soft-tissue facial volume in the aged face and mask contour irregularities and mild skeletal deficiencies in younger patients. Adipose-derived stem cells within the graft provide anti-inflammatory benefits and have been reported to improve overlying dermis quality and scars [16]. Coleman has written extensively on the benefits of fat grafting including skin quality improvement, softening of wrinkles, decreasing pore size and hyperpigmentation, and overall scar quality improvement [17, 18]. Fat grafting has been shown to improve metrics in wound healing, scarring, and postoperative edema [19], the mitigation of which is key to critically analyzing modifications to the facial mask and improving patient satisfaction. Fat grafting also serves to treat pre-existing subclinical facial asymmetry [20], and it can improve aesthetic outcomes with minimal donor site morbidity and cost [21] (Fig. 13.4). This adjunctive procedure has little effect on operative time when combined with other facial aesthetic or orthognathic procedures. The use of fat can provide a blended contour of the chin with the inferior border of the mandible following osseous genioplasty, and it can also correct an excessively deep labiomental crease that can result from bony or alloplastic augmentation [22, 23].

Small-volume facial fat grafting is typically conducted with the use of 3–4 mm liposuction cannulas, either harvested by hand with a syringe or attached to external suction with a trap to collect the harvested graft. The ideal donor site for fat grafting is usually dictated by the patient's individual anatomy, though research has suggested that the lower abdomen and inner thigh may have higher concentrations of fat cells without meaningful difference in adipose cell viability [24]. These sites are easily accessible and possess adequate volume for harvest. While the final graft take can be quite variable in large volumes, the use of small aliquots in a well-vascularized soft tissue envelope of the face is likely to result in 60–70% graft survival [2].

A multitude of techniques have been described to process lipoaspirate. Balancing viability, volume, cost, and efficiency is of key consideration. Centrifugation, Telfa-rolling, gravity filtration, and mesh filtration have all been used with positive reported results. While the processing technique varies based on the surgeon preference, volume, and cost, it is largely accepted that gentle handling and atraumatic treatment of lipoaspirate are the most important components to minimize shear force and maximize cell viability. Our practice is to use gentle Telfa-rolling to process lipoaspirate, before transferring the graft material into 1 cc syringes for injection with a 19-gauge sharp needle [2] (Fig. 13.5).

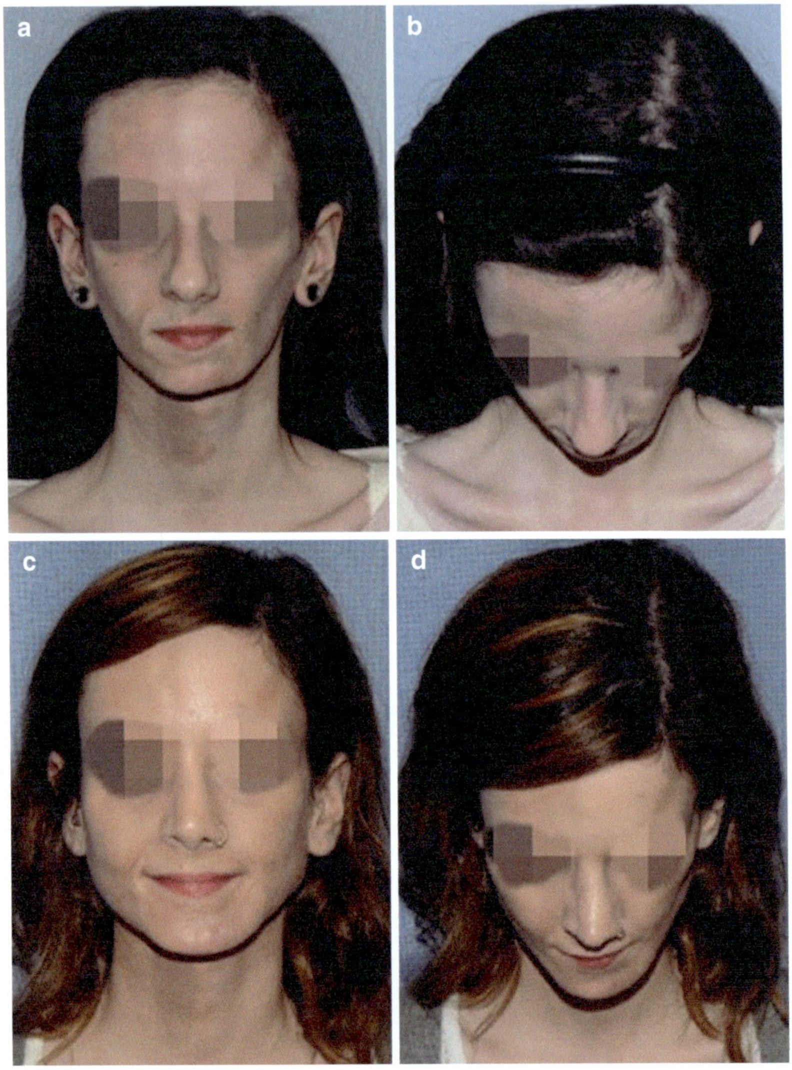

Fig. 13.4 Fat grafting. (**a**–**b**) Preoperative frontal and bird's-eye photographs of a 22-year-old female with scleroderma who presented with significant facial soft tissue atrophy. (**c**–**d**) Postoperative photographs demonstrating restoration of facial soft tissue volume with fat grafting

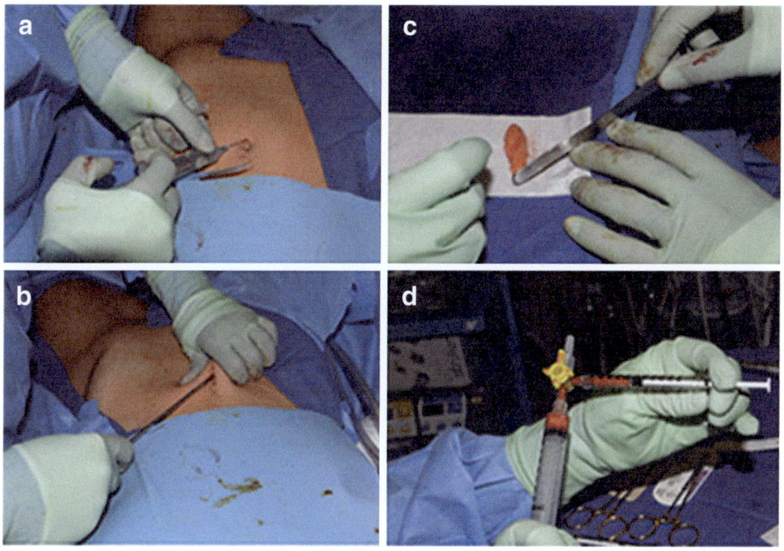

Fig. 13.5 Fat grafting technique. (**a**) Local anesthetic with epinephrine is injected into donor site for a tumescent and hemostatic effect. (**b**) Small stab incision is made, and fat is harvested using a 3 mm or 4 mm Coleman cannula. (**c**) Fat is then gently rolled on Telfa to remove impurities and liquid. (**d**) Fat can then be transferred using a three-way stopcock into 1 cc syringes. Using a 19G needle, the fat can be injected in small aliquots to the desired recipient site

13.4 Buccal Fat Pad Excision

Anatomically, the lower face contour is composed of four elements: the buccal fat pad, masseter muscle, mandible, and subcutaneous fat. The buccal fat pad (BFP) is a rounded trilobed adipose structure with a close relationship with the temporal masticatory space, facial nerve branches, and the parotid duct [25]. The buccal fat pad is unique among the other facial fat compartments in that it straddles both the superficial and deep fat compartments. Patients with an excessive buccal fat pad may complain of an overly rounded, puffy, or "baby-faced" appearance despite being at an appropriate weight, and they may desire more sculpted features [26]. In select patients, judicious buccal fat pad resection enhances the zygomatic prominences, slims the lower facial third, and provides an overall pleasing inverted-triangular contour to the face (Fig. 13.1b). While appropriate candidates for BFP excision are identified based on physical exam and patient aesthetic goals, the procedure is contraindicated in patients with Parry–Romberg Syndrome, wherein BFP atrophy is a well-known clinical sign [27].

While BFP excision can be combined with rhytidectomy and performed extraorally through the same incision, it is more commonly (and more safely) approached intraorally through a maxillary gingivobuccal sulcus incision. After dissection through the buccinator muscle, the fat pad can be exposed, and with gentle external pressure, the exposed herniated portion of the fat pad can be clamped and excised (Fig. 13.1d). Potential complications of BFP excision include hematoma, trismus, infection, facial nerve impairment, parotid duct injury, over-resection, and asymmetry [28, 29].

There is much interest in the role of the buccal fat pad as it relates to facial aging. While Matarasso reported a weak relationship between aging and buccal fat loss [30], more recent studies seem to indicate that the BFP does volumetrically diminish over time, especially after the age of 20 [31]. In a series of 22 buccal fat pad dissections, Zhang et al. demonstrated that the intermediate lobe of the BFP was well developed in children and smaller and more poorly defined in adults [32]. The hollowing of the nasojugal fold and tear troughs noted with age-related descent of the fat compartments is in part attributable to the volume loss of the buccal extension of the BFP [33]. These studies suggest that the BFP does change with aging, and for that reason, caution is recommended in performing aggressive fat pad resection in younger patients as it may have negative long-term effects.

13.5 Conclusions

While orthognathic surgery can improve facial balance, patients may achieve optimal aesthetic outcomes with the use of more minor ancillary procedures to augment or restore soft tissue or bony volume or, alternatively, judicious subcutaneous or fat pad resection to provide a more sculpted, elevated look. These procedures are safe, effective, and can be quickly performed with appropriate planning.

References

1. Rosen HM. Evolution of a surgical philosophy in orthognathic surgery. Plast Reconstr Surg. 2017;139(4):978–90.
2. Steinbacher DM. Alloplastic facial augmentation in aesthetic rhinoplasty and orthognathic surgery. Hoboken: Wiley Blackwell; 2019. p. 559–72.
3. Steinbacher DM. Chin and submental aesthetics, in aesthetic orthognathic surgery and rhinoplasty. Hoboken: Wiley Blackwell; 2019.
4. White JB, Dufresne CR. Management and avoidance of complications in chin augmentation. Aesthet Surg J. 2011;31(6):634–42.
5. Kelly JP, Malik S, Stucki-McCormick SU. Tender swelling of the chin 40 years after genioplasty. J Oral Maxillofac Surg. 2000;58(2):203–6.
6. Yaremchuk MJ. Facial skeletal reconstruction using porous polyethylene implants. Plast Reconstr Surg. 2003;111(6):1818–27.
7. Yaremchuk MJ. Secondary malar implant surgery. Plast Reconstr Surg. 2008;121(2):620–8.
8. Zide BM, Pfeifer TM, Longaker MT. Chin surgery: I. Augmentation—the allures and the alerts. Plast Reconstr Surg. 1999;104(6):1843–53. discussion 1861–2
9. Hsieh TY, et al. Alloplastic facial implants. Facial Plast Surg. 2021;37(6):741–50.
10. Wrzosek MK, et al. Comparison of time required for traditional versus virtual orthognathic surgery treatment planning. Int J Oral Maxillofac Surg. 2016;45(9):1065–9.
11. French KEM, et al. Outcomes and complications associated with malar onlays: literature review and case series of 119 implants. Br J Oral Maxillofac Surg. 2020;58(9):1110–5.
12. Doddamani GM, Swathi PV, Tan KFH. Assessment of anterior malar projection using visual photographs and lateral cephalograms: a comparative study. J Orthod Sci. 2018;7:15.
13. Goldsmith D, Horowitz A, Orentlicher G. Facial skeletal augmentation using custom facial implants. Atlas Oral Maxillofac Surg Clin North Am. 2012;20(1):119–34.
14. Eppley BL. Mandibular Angle Implants. Facial Plast Surg. 2019;35(2):158–63.
15. Thomas MA, Yaremchuk MJ. Masseter muscle reattachment after mandibular angle surgery. Aesthet Surg J. 2009;29(6):473–6.
16. Lisa A, et al. The use of autologous fat grafting for treatment of scar tissue and scar-related conditions: a systematic review. Plast Reconstr Surg. 2016;138(6):1076e–7e.
17. Coleman SR. Facial augmentation with structural fat grafting. Clin Plast Surg. 2006;33(4):567–77.
18. Coleman SR. Structural fat grafting: more than a permanent filler. Plast Reconstr Surg. 2006;118(3 Suppl):108s–20s.
19. Cabrejo R, et al. Does fat grafting influence postoperative edema in orthognathic surgery? J Craniofac Surg. 2017;28(8):1906–10.
20. Wang YC, et al. Orthognathic surgery with simultaneous autologous fat transfer for correction of facial asymmetry. Plast Reconstr Surg. 2017;139(3):693–700.
21. Iyengar RJ, et al. Fat grafting in orthognathic surgery. J Craniofac Surg. 2019;30(3):639–43.
22. Rohrich RJ, Sanniec K, Afrooz PN. Autologous fat grafting to the chin: a useful adjunct in complete aesthetic facial rejuvenation. Plast Reconstr Surg. 2018;142(4):921–5.
23. Wang Q, Guo X, Wang J. Autogenous fat grafting for chin augmentation: a preliminarily clinical study of cosmetic outcome. J Craniofac Surg. 2015;26(7):e625–7.
24. Padoin AV, et al. Sources of processed lipoaspirate cells: influence of donor site on cell concentration. Plast Reconstr Surg. 2008;122(2):614–8.
25. Moura LB, et al. Buccal fat pad removal to improve facial aesthetics: an established technique? Med Oral Patol Oral Cir Bucal. 2018;23(4):e478–84.
26. Davis B, Serra M. Buccal fat pad reduction. In: StatPearls. Treasure Island: StatPearls Publishing; 2022.
27. Oyama T, et al. Bilayer reconstruction for parry-romberg syndrome: using a free circumflex scapular artery-based adipofascial flap for both the

buccal fat pad and subcutaneous fat. Ann Plast Surg. 2011;67(4):372–5.

28. Traboulsi-Garet B, et al. Buccal fat pad excision for cheek refinement: a systematic review. Med Oral Patol Oral Cir Bucal. 2021;26(4):e474–81.
29. Pimentel T, et al. Management of complications related to removal of the buccal fat pad. J Craniofac Surg. 2021;32(3):e238–40.
30. Matarasso A. Managing the buccal fat pad. Aesthet Surg J. 2006;26(3):330–6.
31. Rohrich RJ, et al. The role of the buccal fat pad in facial aesthetic surgery. Plast Reconstr Surg. 2021;148(2):334–8.
32. Zhang HM, et al. Anatomical structure of the buccal fat pad and its clinical adaptations. Plast Reconstr Surg. 2002;109(7):2509–18; discussion 2519–20.
33. Gierloff M, et al. Aging changes of the midfacial fat compartments: a computed tomographic study. Plast Reconstr Surg. 2012;129(1):263–73.

14 Peroperative Surgical Management and Recommendations

Adaia Valls Ontañón and Orion-Luiz Haas-Junior

14.1 Introduction

Preoperative management of the patient, along with specific recommendations, improve the final outcomes and patient experience during the procedure.

On one hand, the establishment of a good and trusting professional (team)–patient relationship is of uppermost importance. In this regard, it is useful to explain the planned procedures in depth and indicate the expected results and eventual complications to the patient and his/her relatives. Keeping close contact through telephone or videoconference support during the postoperative period, with frequent follow-up visits, is also useful. Moreover, coordination and fluent contact between professionals is also important in order to avoid conflicting messages for the patient that could make him/her feel insecure. This should start from the beginning of the treatment plan.

On the other hand, all steps and recommendations in the preoperative and postoperative periods must be systematized by the healthcare team to streamline the process, so that the patient can enjoy as much comfort as possible and avoid any concerns with the bureaucracy of admission or with the need to secure support after surgery. The following list of key points summarizes the daily protocol of the authors.

14.2 Preoperative Assessment

14.2.1 Patient Systemic Health

During the first visit, evaluation of the systemic condition of the patient, with an assessment of his/her past medical history, is paramount. When relevant comorbidities are present, these must be controlled and should not contraindicate surgical intervention. Otherwise, the procedure should be deferred until control of the underlying disease condition has been achieved, always bearing in mind that orthognathic surgery is an elective procedure. In addition, preoperatively, we routinely request a series of laboratory tests (complete blood count, platelet count, coagulation parameters, urea, creatinine, and fasting blood glucose), imaging tests (thoracic radiography in patients with a history of chronic obstructive pulmonary disease or smoking), and an electrocardiogram (in patients with mild heart disease or women over 40 years of age).

A. Valls Ontañón (✉)
Department of Oral and Maxillofacial Surgery, International University of Catalonia, Barcelona, Spain
e-mail: avalls@uic.es

O.-L. Haas-Junior
Department of Oral and Maxillofacial Surgery, Hospital São Lucas – Pontifícia Universidade Católica do Rio Grande do Sul, Porto Alegre, Brazil

Blanc Hospital, Porto Alegre, Brazil

F. Hernández-Alfaro, A. Valls Ontañón (eds.), *Orthofacial Surgery*,
https://doi.org/10.1007/978-3-031-76185-0_14

14.2.2 Temporomandibular Joint Evaluation

Similarly, temporomandibular joint morphological and functional assessment should be carried out before starting any orthodontic surgical treatment [1].

Morphologically, the following aspects are evaluated by cone-beam computed tomography (CBCT): overall relevant anatomical structures, cortical bone of the mandibular condyles to rule out signs of osteoarthrosis such as surface destruction or osteophytes, and assessment of possible condylar resorption or hyperplasia (Fig. 14.1) [2, 3].

Clinically, the patient is examined for intra-articular symptoms, dislocation of the joint disc, or difficulty opening the mouth.

If any disease or anomaly is detected, its management should be discussed first, and the patient should be informed about the impact of orthognathic surgery upon it.

14.2.3 Dental Occlusion

Of all the analyses, preoperative dental occlusion is the aspect which will tell us whether a patient is fit to undergo orthognathic surgery or not [4]. Working together with the orthodontist, we will define the optimal timing of the surgical procedure and which timing protocol should be adopted (surgery first, surgery early, surgery late, surgery last, or surgery only) [4–7].

Then, having confirmed (by both the orthodontist and the surgeon) that the dental occlusion of the patient is satisfactory and stable for the postoperative period, surgery will be scheduled.

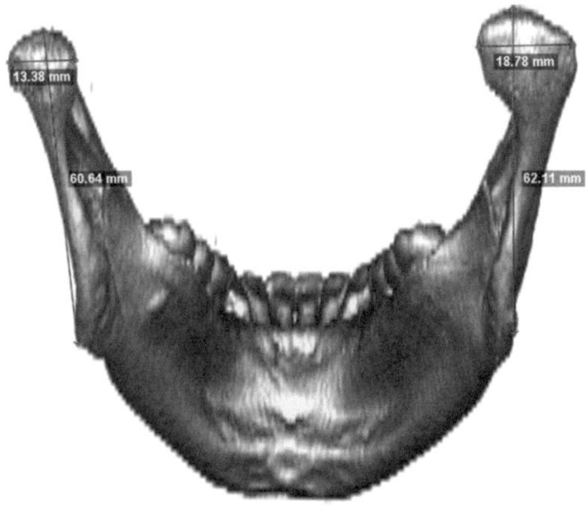

Fig. 14.1 CBCT evaluation of mandibular asymmetry secondary to condyle hyperplasia. Proportional condylectomy can thus be planned

14.2.4 Preoperative Recommendations

During the preoperative period, a number of recommendations are made, and a comprehensive diagnostic checklist should be administered to ascertain whether the patient is fit to undergo orthognathic surgery in the coming days:

- During preoperative orthodontic treatment and before surgery, all patients are instructed on *strict dental hygiene* measures following the modified Bass technique [8], and 1 week before surgery, all patients undergo *professional dental cleaning*.
- Before obtaining the surgical planning records (a single CBCT scan) (iCAT, Imaging Sciences International, Hatfield, PA, USA) of the head of the patient, with intraoral surface scanning of the dental arches using the Lava Scan ST scanner (3 M ESPE, Ann Arbor, MI, USA), the orthodontist is contacted in order to indicate the date for obtaining the *registration records*. From then on, the orthodontist is asked to not perform any additional orthodontic movements.
- Before surgery, the orthodontist should place a heavy (0.19″ × 0.21″ or 0.19″ × 0.25″) *nickel–titanium rectangular passive arch-wire*, ensure brackets' and bands' stability, and place ligature hooks into the arch for surgical intermaxillary fixation. When maxillary segmentation is required, the steel arch should be cut at the level of the segmentation (Fig. 14.2) and ideally with previous separation of the dental roots (Fig. 14.3). However, nowadays orthognathic surgery can be carried out without braces or arch-wires or hooks,

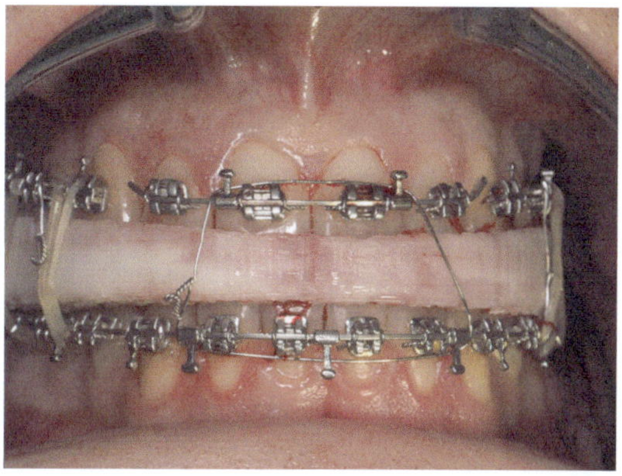

Fig. 14.2 Intraoperative view showing bilateral cut of the steel arch at the level of the maxillary segmentation

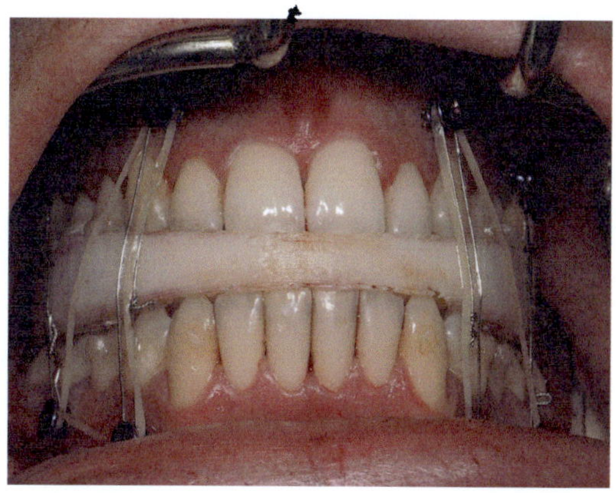

Fig. 14.4 Intermaxillary fixation screws for intraoperative intermaxillary fixation and postoperative elastic guidance or orthodontic anchorage

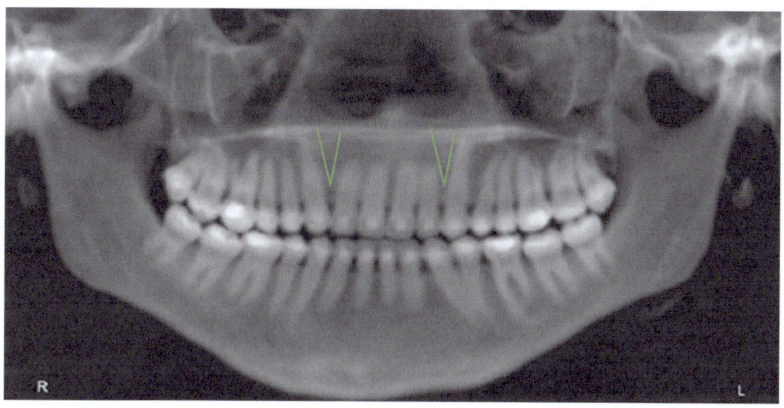

Fig. 14.3 Panoramic radiograph showing separation of dental roots at the level of the segmentation via orthodontics

since *intermaxillary fixation screws* can be placed intraoperatively just before the surgical procedure. It is useful in cases following the surgery-only strategy or using aligners or lingual orthodontics (Fig. 14.4).

- Three days before surgery, the patient starts using a *nasal corticosteroid spray* (Nasonex®) every 8 h, which reduces nasal mucosa swelling and irritation, and thus facilitates nasal floor dissection and diminishes its bleeding during surgery [9].

14.3 Intraoperative Recommendations

- In patients undergoing general anesthesia, nasotracheal intubation and a *pharyngeal tamponade* are placed.
- Intraoperative-controlled *hypotension* is recommended [10].
- Minimally invasive surgical techniques as well as limiting the surgery time will improve the outcomes and the postoperative period.
- As adjuvant measures, all patients receive intraoperative *corticosteroids* (methylprednisolone, 15 mg/kg iv), *antifibrinolytic* treatment (tranexamic acid, 15 mg/kg iv), *antiemetic* medication (ondansetron, 4 mg iv), *antibiotic* therapy (amoxicillin-clavulanic acid, 2 g iv; in the case of beta-lactamase allergy, clindamycin, 600 mg iv and gentamycin, 240 mg), *gastric protection* (ranitidine, 50 mg iv), *analgesics* (paracetamol, 1 g iv, dexketoprofen, 50 mg iv, diclofenac, 75 mg im), and ketamine at sub-anesthetic doses (20 mg iv in induction and 40 mg iv in slow administration during surgery) [11].
- Even when a pharyngeal tamponade is placed, *gastric aspiration* is recommended, since blood in the stomach is very irritative and may induce nausea and vomiting.

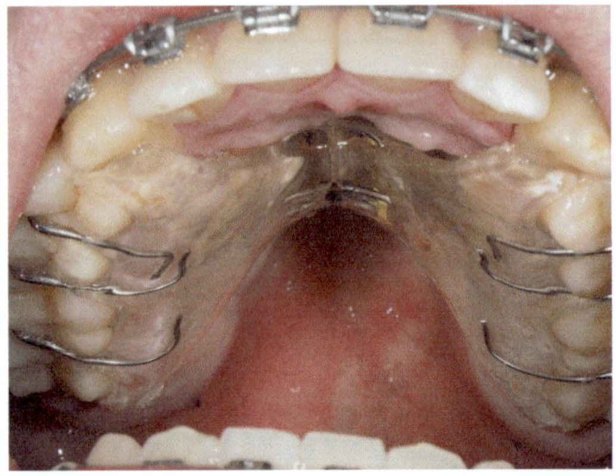

Fig. 14.5 A removable palatal Hawley plate fixed with Adams hooks to the teeth is left in place in patients undergoing maxillary segmentation in order to avoid skeletal relapse, which furthermore can be activated if further maxillary expansion is required postoperatively

14.4 Postoperative Care

The following protocol is adopted in the postoperative period to assist in prompt recovery from the first 24 h of hospitalization up to 1 month after orthognathic surgery.

14.4.1 Immediate Postoperative Recommendations

- In patients undergoing maxillary segmentation, a removable palatal Hawley plate fixed with Adams hooks to the teeth is left in place in order to avoid skeletal relapse (Fig. 14.5), which furthermore can be activated if further maxillary expansion is required postoperatively.
- *Intermaxillary elastic fixation* is placed to guide occlusion at the end of surgery after pharyngeal tamponade removal and before patient extubation. These intermaxillary elastics exert little force, serving only to guide the muscles of mastication toward their new position over a 1 month period after surgery. Our routine practice is to use guiding box elastics (Fig. 14.6). The patient is instructed to change them at meals after the first week.
- Anti-inflammatory and analgesic agents and antibiotics are administered intravenously while the patient is in hospital. Antiemetics are also prescribed as needed. After discharge, the same medication regimen is continued orally.
- All patients wear a *closed-circuit cold mask* (facial mask Hilotherm® GmbH; Argenbühl, Germany) at 17 °C during hospital admission. It provides comfort and relieves pain by reducing nerve transmission in the region and preventing the progression of edema and hematoma by decreasing the capacity for fluid buildup within the soft tissues of the face [12–14] (Fig. 14.7). After hospital discharge, the patient is instructed to continue applying an ice pack to the face for up to 48 h.

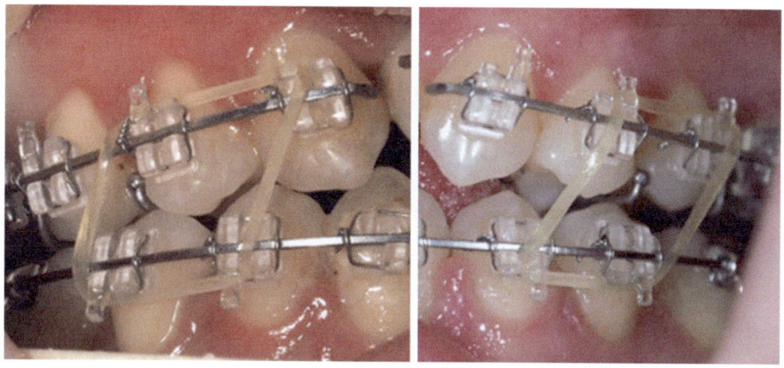

Fig. 14.6 Intermaxillary elastic fixation to guide muscles to the new occlusion using guiding box elastics. Its direction might depend on the muscular forces

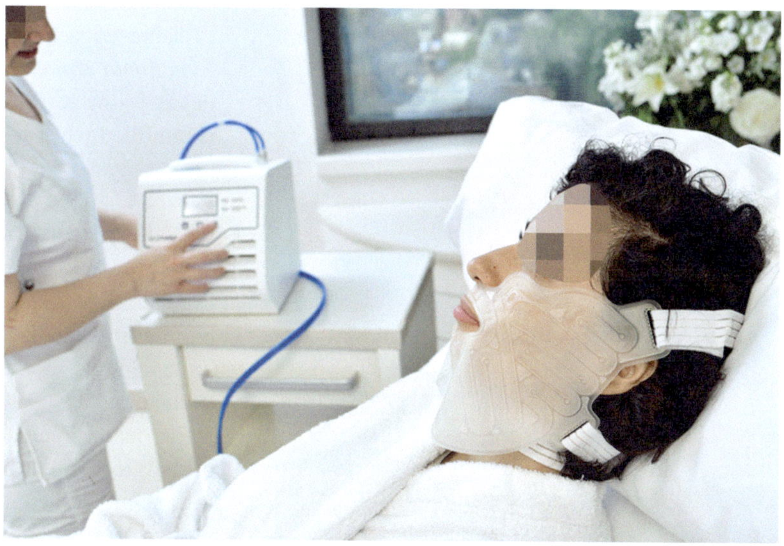

Fig. 14.7 Cold therapy using a closed-circuit cold mask (17 °C) is prescribed during hospital admission

- Patients start *oral* liquids and soft diet *tolerance* 6 h after surgery. The use of a glass and spoon are recommended from minute one. Feeding syringes can be used when necessary, but sucking with drinking straws is not allowed.
- *Facial and cervical lymphatic drainage* is performed a few hours after surgery and/or the day after by experienced personnel (Fig. 14.8). Implementing this treatment in the immediate postoperative period accelerates the drainage of facial edema by stimulating the lymphatic system and contributing to regional blood circulation. The benefits of massage include facilitating early mandibular mobility, which allows the patient to open and close the mouth soon after surgery, and re-establishing normal facial movements.
- Then, a *kinesiological tape* is placed over the operated area to accelerate drainage of the tissue reaction (Fig. 14.9) [15].
- The patient should start *walking* as soon as possible, since it reduces swelling, improves the mood state, and reduces the recovery period.
- The day after surgery, the patient undergoes *oral cleansing with 0.12% chlorhexidine* and is instructed on dental hygiene with a soft brush for the external dental surface (also internal if there is enough mouth opening), 0.12% chlorhexidine mouth rinses, and a water jet (Lacer®).
- *Nasal cleansing irrigations* are made with mild cold saline solution (or Rinhomer) (kept in the fridge). Blowing is forbidden.
- *Sleeping in a 45° position* (two pillows) is indicated to facilitate breathing and avoid facial edema.

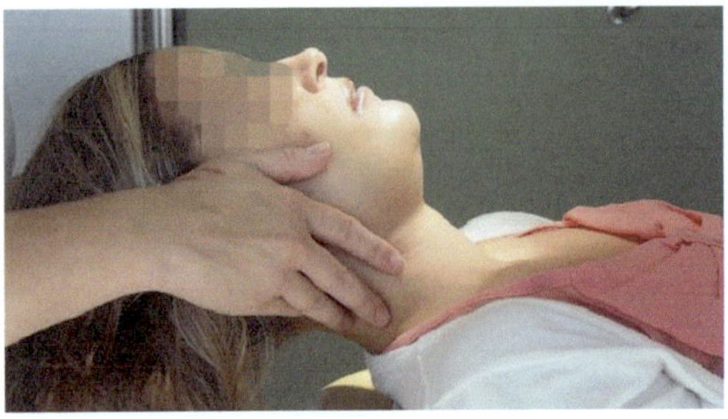

Fig. 14.8 Facial and cervical lymphatic drainage accelerates the drainage of facial edema by stimulating the lymphatic system and contributing to regional blood circulation

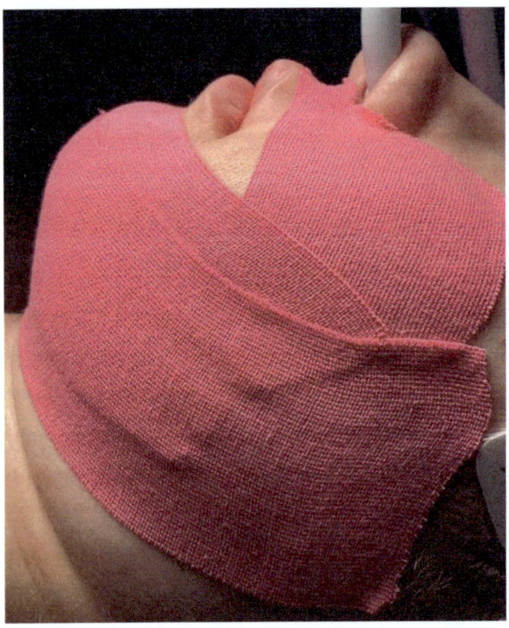

Fig. 14.9 A kinesiological tape is placed over the operated area to accelerate drainage of the tissue reaction

14.4.2 Home Postoperative Recommendations

- A liquid *diet* is recommended during the first week, and thereafter a soft diet is followed for 3 months.
- At 1 week of follow-up, the patient is instructed on the *"five-step procedure"* for elastic removal, with mouth-opening exercises (10 times), eating a soft diet, strict oral hygiene, and guiding elastic placement. Mouth-opening exercises may be added gradually:
  - First week: Mouth opening and closing without straining. Facial mimics and speaking may be helpful.
  - Second week: Gentle stretching of the jaw muscles by pressing fingers between the back teeth on either side, as well as moving of the jaw from side to side and from back to front.
  - Third week: Gentle opening of a wooden clothes peg placed in the lateral sides of the mouth. Once maximum central opening is achieved, a second peg can be added.
- *Functional training* using light guiding elastics is followed for 1 month, and the position is modified when required.

14.5 Key Points

- Preoperative assessment of the oral cavity, temporomandibular joint, and systemic health is essential, apart from the dentofacial evaluation.
- Strict dental hygiene is mandatory during all the surgical and orthodontic processes.
- Intraoperative controlled hypotension and proper medication, minimally invasive surgical techniques, as well as limiting the surgery time, will improve the outcomes and postoperative period.
- Intermaxillary elastic fixation is placed to guide occlusion at the end of surgery.
- At 1 week of follow-up, the patient is instructed on the "five-step procedure" for elastic removal, with mouth-opening exercises (10 times), eating a soft diet, strict oral hygiene, and guiding elastic placement.

References

1. Mendez-Manjon I, Guijarro-Martinez R, Valls-Ontañón A, Hernandez-Alfaro F. Early changes in condylar position after mandibular advancement: a three-dimensional analysis. Int J Oral Maxillofac Surg. 2016;45(6):787–92.

2. Méndez-Manjón I, Haas OLJ, Guijarro-Martínez R, Belle de Oliveira R, Valls-Ontañón A, Hernández-Alfaro F. Semi-automated three-dimensional condylar reconstruction. J Craniofac Surg. 2019;30(8):2555–9.
3. Larheim TA, Abrahamsson A-K, Kristensen M, Arvidsson LZ. Temporomandibular joint diagnostics using CBCT. Dentomaxillofac Radiol. 2015;44(1):20140235.
4. Hernandez-Alfaro F, Guijarro-Martinez R. On a definition of the appropriate timing for surgical intervention in orthognathic surgery. Int J Oral Maxillofac Surg. 2014;43(7):846–55.
5. Hernández-Alfaro F, Guijarro-Martínez R, Molina-Coral A, Badía-Escriche C. "Surgery first" in bimaxillary orthognathic surgery. J Oral Maxillofac Surg [Internet]. 2011;69(6):e201–7. https://doi.org/10.1016/j.joms.2011.01.010.
6. Peiró-Guijarro MA, Guijarro-Martínez R, Hernández-Alfaro F. Surgery first in orthognathic surgery: a systematic review of the literature. Am J Orthod Dentofacial Orthop. 2016;149(4):448–62.
7. Hernandez-Alfaro F, Guijarro-Martinez R, Peiro-Guijarro MA. Surgery first in orthognathic surgery: what have we learned? A comprehensive workflow based on 45 consecutive cases. J Oral Maxillofac Surg. 2014;72(2):376–90.
8. Poyato M, Segura J, Bullón P. Comparison of modified bass technique with normal toothbrushing practices for efficacy in supragingival plaque removal. Int J Dent Hyg. 2003;1(2):110–4.
9. Benninger MS, Ahmad N, Marple BF. The safety of intranasal steroids. Otolaryngol Head Neck Surg. 2003;129(6):739–50.
10. Kouz K, Hoppe P, Briesenick L, Saugel B. Intraoperative hypotension: pathophysiology, clinical relevance, and therapeutic approaches. Indian J Anaesth. 2020;64(2):90–6.
11. Molins-Ballabriga G, Hernández-Alfaro F, Giralt-Hernando M, Valls-Ontañón A. Multimodal analgesia in orthognathic surgery. J Oral Maxillofac Anesth. 2022;1:20.
12. Glass GE, Waterhouse N, Shakib K. Hilotherapy for the management of perioperative pain and swelling in facial surgery: a systematic review and meta-analysis. Br J Oral Maxillofac Surg. 2016;54(8):851–6.
13. Bates AS, Knepil GJ. Systematic review and meta-analysis of the efficacy of hilotherapy following oral and maxillofacial surgery. Int J Oral Maxillofac Surg [Internet]. 2016;45(1):110–7. https://doi.org/10.1016/j.ijom.2015.08.983.
14. El-Karmi A, Hassfeld S, Bonitz L. Development of swelling following orthognathic surgery at various cooling temperatures by means of hilotherapy–a clinical, prospective, monocentric, single-blinded, randomised study. J Cranio-Maxillofac Surg [Internet]. 2018;46(9):1401–7. https://doi.org/10.1016/j.jcms.2018.01.012.
15. Ristow O, Pautke C, Kehl V, Koerdt S, Schwärzler K, Hahnefeld L, et al. Influence of kinesiologic tape on postoperative swelling, pain and trismus after zygomatico-orbital fractures. J Cranio-Maxillofacial Surg [Internet]. 2014;42(5):469–76. https://doi.org/10.1016/j.jcms.2013.05.043.

15 Airway and Skeletal Surgery

Adaia Valls Ontañón

15.1 Introduction

Obstructive sleep apnea (OSA) is a sleep-related breathing disorder characterized by respiratory pauses secondary to partial (hypopnea) or complete (apnea) obstruction of the pharyngeal airway (PA), with a duration of at least 10 s [1]. The PA is occluded due to a loss of muscle tone of the PA dilator muscles during sleep, which leads to narrowing or total obstruction of the PA [1, 2]. As a result, there are repetitive oxygen desaturation episodes with snoring, unrefreshing sleep, fatigue, and excessive daytime sleepiness. Systemic arterial hypertension and heart failure may subsequently develop, with a significant increase in mortality risk. Overall, OSA may also have a social impact in terms of poor quality of life, days of work lost, and traffic accidents [1].

It is estimated that OSA affects 5–20% of the general adult population, though some authors report figures of up to 26% [3, 4]. Nevertheless, the statistics show that over 50% of all cases go undiagnosed [3]. The disorder is 3 times more common in men than in women and more prevalent in patients with dentofacial deformities (DFDs), retrusive jaw patterns being the most affected [3]. Young patients with underlying maxillary or mandibular hypoplasia tend to suffer from mild OSA, which is clinically silent, since they are not aware of the disorder [5]. However, from the age of 30, and over time, the volume of the PA (PAV) decreases, since the pharyngeal musculature loses tone [6]. Thus, patients with an underlying hypoplastic DFD will probably reduce their upper airway (UA) volume and therefore develop more severe OSA over the years.

Continuous positive airway pressure (CPAP) is considered the gold standard treatment in this regard. However, since CPAP non-adherence rates of 46–86% have been reported [7], different alternative surgical treatments have been proposed to expand the PA, such as uvulopalatopharyngoplasty, hyoid suspension, or hyothyroidopexy, with low success rates, and the results moreover do not hold up over time [8]. On the other hand, tonsillectomy and adenoidectomy are indicated procedures for children with hypertrophy of these organs [9].

Since Guilleminault et al. [10] first described maxillomandibular advancement (MMA) as an effective treatment for patients with OSA [10], several studies have confirmed its benefits. Many publications have demonstrated that new positioning of the muscles attached to the jaws and pharyngeal walls in the context of MMA results in enlargement of the PA and, consequently, a decrease in the apnea–hypopnea index (AHI). Some authors have concluded that the efficacy of

A. Valls Ontañón (✉)
Department of Oral and Maxillofacial Surgery, International University of Catalonia, Barcelona, Spain
e-mail: avalls@uic.es

F. Hernández-Alfaro, A. Valls Ontañón (eds.), *Orthofacial Surgery*,
https://doi.org/10.1007/978-3-031-76185-0_15

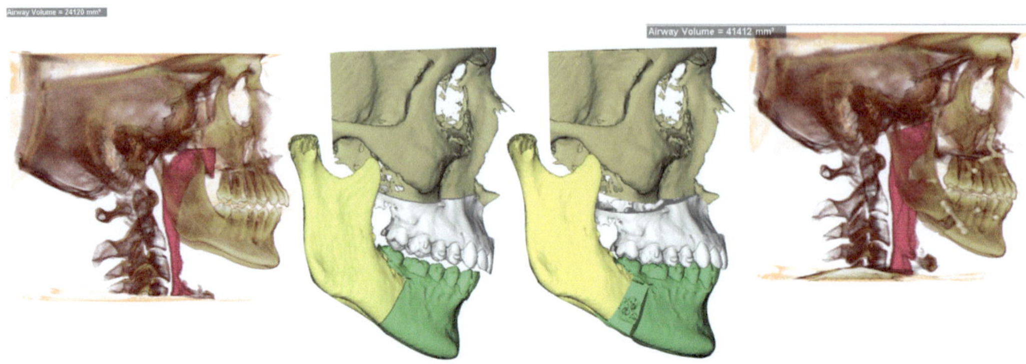

Fig. 15.1 Impact of widening of the maxillomandibular framework on upper airway volume

MMA in patients with an underlying dentofacial deformity is equivalent to that of CPAP use over the long term [7] (Fig. 15.1). Thus, orthognathic surgery (OS) is currently considered to be a first-line option for treating patients with moderate and severe OSA (over 15 episodes/hour [e/h]) [11], with a high surgical success rate of 87.5% [2] (success being defined as a final AHI threshold of <20 e/h, with a reduction of 50%) [7]. However, there is a lack of evidence supporting the management of mild OSA (5–15 e/h) through OS. According to our experience, these patients also benefit from a reduction of the number of apnea/hypopnea episodes following OS, due to the UA enlargement achieved, with an OSA cure rate of 50%.

15.2 Patient Selection

As previously mentioned, orthognathic surgery is indicated for OSA patients with an underlying dentofacial deformity amenable to surgery. The following dentofacial morphological characteristics are more prone to cause OSA: class II malocclusion patients, a biretrusive facial profile, steep occlusal plane, and/or a narrow palate.

On the other hand, mandibular advancement devices are reserved for non-obese patients with mild-to-moderate OSA refractory to, or non-compliant with, continuous positive airway pressure, and for patients who are not candidates for surgery due to health reasons, and also as a prognostic element in eventual orthognathic surgery. If the mandibular advancement device proves effective, surgery will be even more so.

15.3 OSA Diagnosis and Monitoring in Daily Practice

In patients who come to our consultation and in whom an obstructive apnea problem is suspected, daytime sleepiness is tested using the Epworth Sleepiness Scale (ESS) [12]. This instrument is a reasonable predictor of OSA risk and consists of a simple self-administered questionnaire. If the scale proves positive, polysomnography (PSG) or home sleep apnea testing is requested [13].

Polysomnography is considered the gold standard for diagnosing and monitoring OSA [4, 14]. It records brain activity, breathing, heart rate, muscle activity, snoring, and blood oxygen levels while resting/sleeping and during repeated episodes of PA obstruction. The measurements are based on the AHI. Since PSG requires hospital admission during one night, home sleep apnea testing devices can be used for the diagnosis of uncomplicated OSA in adults (as indicated by the American Academy of Sleep Medicine guidelines) [4, 14]. However, standard sleep channels such as the electroencephalogram (EEG) are not monitored by these home devices [4]. In the same line, both tools (ESS and PSG) are used to monitor OSA evolution over time or to evaluate the effectiveness of eventual treatment [4].

Nonetheless, the overall complexity of patients with OSA calls for a multidisciplinary team consisting of a primary care physician, pulmonologist, neurophysiologist, ear, nose and throat specialist, maxillofacial surgeon, orthodontist (and other dental professionals), anesthesiologist, medical rehabilitator, and physiotherapist, among others.

It should be highlighted that other causes of OSA should be evaluated and treated appropriately if possible before DFD surgical treatment, such as overweight, smoking, alcohol abuse, or the presence of central apnea, among other conditions. In cases where surgical effectiveness is doubtful, mandibular advancement devices—apart from being an option for treating mild-to-moderate OSA with better patient compliance than with CPAP [7]—are also useful in deciding which surgical mandibular advancement strategy in the context of OSA is indicated [11].

15.4 Upper Airway Analysis

Airway anatomy is carefully evaluated in all patients undergoing OS, and particularly in cases of OSA. For this purpose, a cone-beam computed tomography (CBCT) study is carried out preoperatively, and a specific 3D software (Dolphin Imaging, version 11.0, Chatsworth, CA, USA) is used to identify the level of the minimal cross-sectional area (mCSA, mm^2) and other airway constriction points and to measure total pharyngeal airway volume (PAV), as well as the naso-, oro-, and hypopharyngeal volumes (mm^3) in particular [15] (Fig. 15.2). Cephalometry allows us to measure the posterior pharyngeal airway but does not afford a three-dimensional (3D) assessment, which is relevant in cases of asymmetries or severe hypoplasia.

Considering where the airway constriction points are located, and taking into account that the estimated mean mCSA and PAV measurements in the healthy population without OSA are 138 mm^2 [16] and 13,200 mm^3 [6], respectively, conclusions can be drawn from the patient airway morphology and volume, allowing us to decide which skeletal movements are required in order to improve the underlying airway constriction condition (Fig. 15.3).

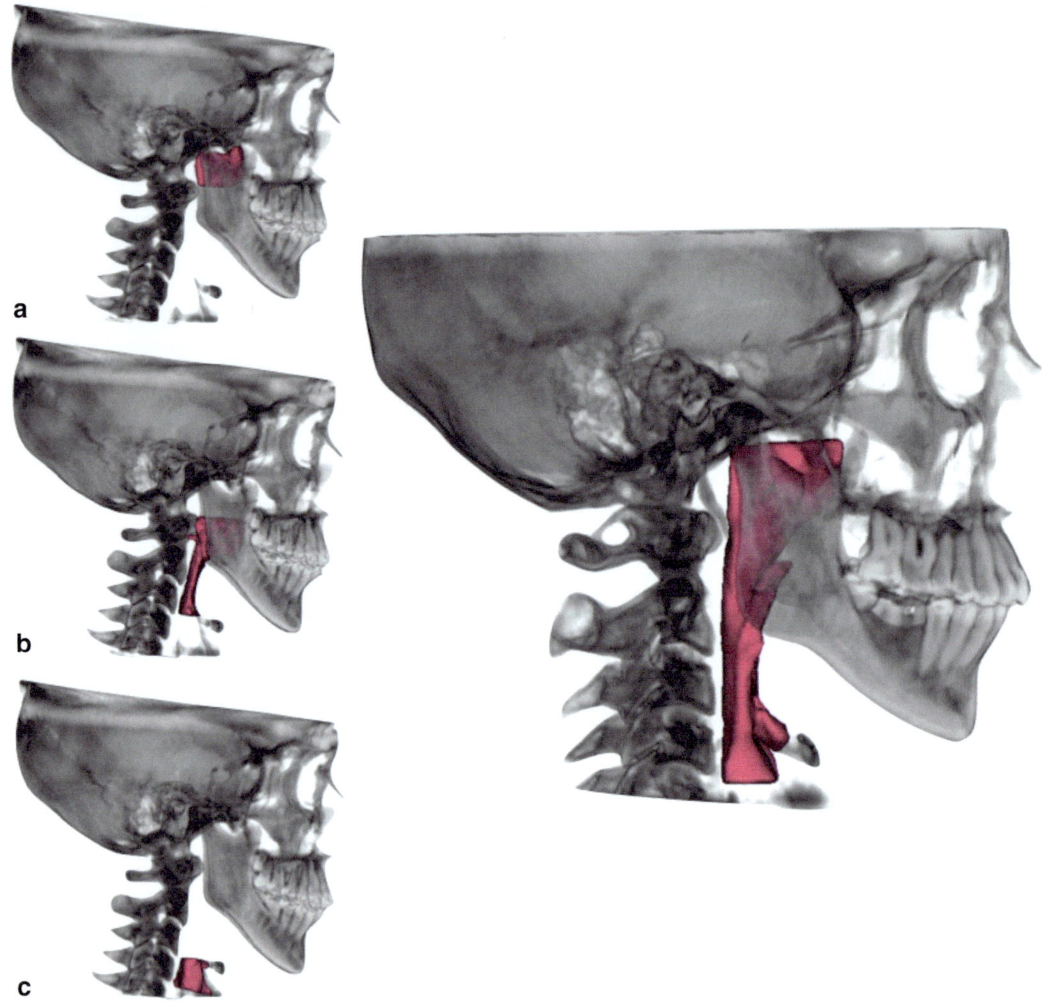

Fig. 15.2 Total pharyngeal airway volume (3D) measurement, and specifically: (**a**) nasopharynx; (**b**) oropharynx; and (**c**) hypopharynx volumes

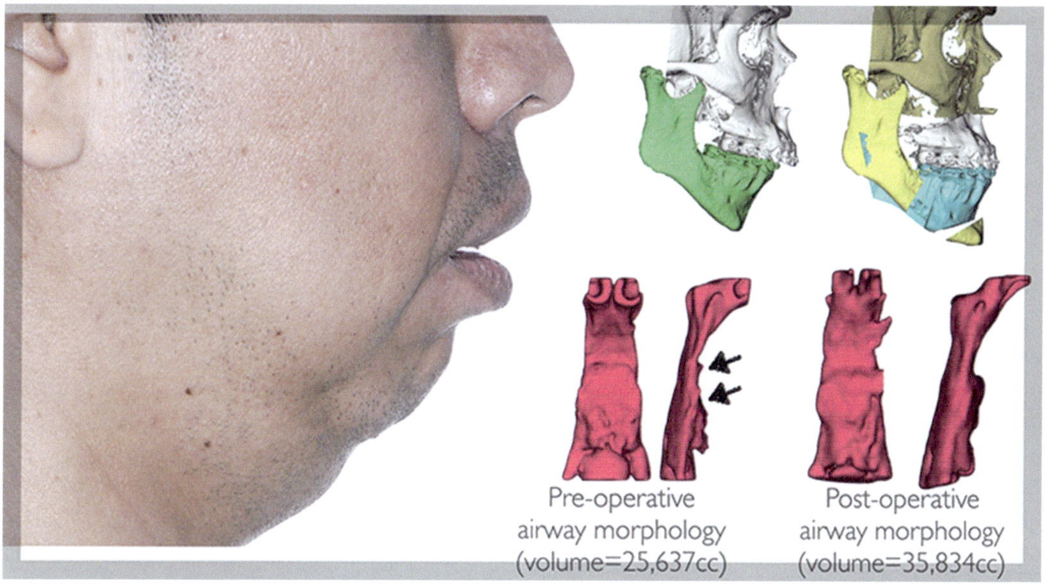

Fig. 15.3 Effect of the lack of skeletal support upon the upper airway, with the constriction points of the airway in the initial (preoperative) situation. Orthognathic surgery with advancement and counterclockwise movement of the maxillomandibular complex and advancement genioplasty enlarges the upper airway and resolves constriction points

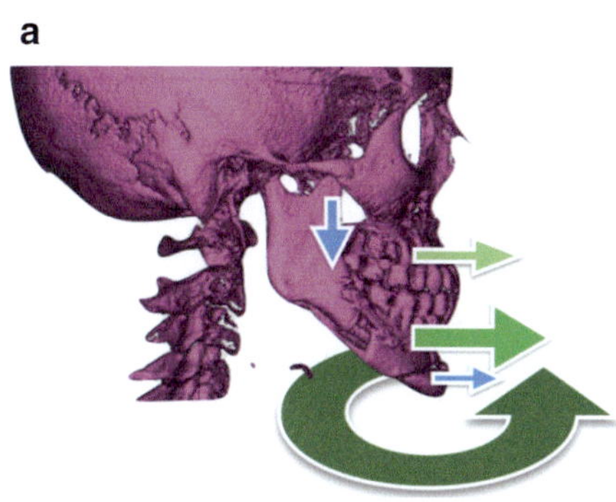

Fig. 15.4 Impact of type and direction of surgical movements upon the upper pharyngeal airway: (**a**) counterclockwise rotation and advancement provide the maximum enlargement, (**b**) while setback and downward movements are detrimental

15.5 Surgical Planning in OSA Patients

Classically, a mean MMA of 10–12 mm has been described as the standard treatment for managing adult patients with moderate-to-severe OSA [2, 10]. However, it has now been widely proven in the literature that other skeletal movements, such as maxillomandibular counterclockwise rotation (CCW), enlarge the PAV even more and therefore further improve AHI [17]. Similarly, it has been broadly demonstrated that framework-widening bimaxillary surgeries achieve larger increases in PAV when compared with single-jaw surgeries [15] (Fig. 15.4).

As previously mentioned, we use the upper incisor to soft-tissue plane (UI-STP) surgical planning protocol or the so-called Barcelona line reference [18], which mainly entails forward projection and CCW rotation of the maxillomandibular framework regardless of the initial occlusal problem (Angle's classification) [19]. Such maxillomandibular complex broadening is consistent with the OS movements required for PA enlargement to treat OSA, as reported in the literature [11, 15]. Thus, in our patients (using the UI-STP surgical planning protocol) [18, 20], a mean PAV increase of 42% ($p < 0.05$) is obtained in bimaxillary surgeries, versus 25.6% ($p < 0.05$) in single maxillary surgeries, and 24.7% ($p < 0.05$) in single mandibular surgeries. Specifically, certain surgical movements following our UI-STP surgical planning protocol favor subregional PAV gain (with statistical significance): maxillary CCW rotation at the nasopharynx ($r = 0.045$, $p < 0.05$), mandibular CCW rotation at the oropharynx ($t = 0.013$, $p < 0.05$), centering of the maxilla at the oropharynx, and sagittal mandibular advancement at the hypopharynx (Mann-Whitney U-test = 0.012, $p < 0.05$). Total PAV is mainly influenced by maxillary and mandibular CCW rotation (Kruskal-Wallis test = 0.032, $p < 0.05$) and centering of the mandible ($t = 0.049$, $p < 0.05$) [15].

Similarly, chin advancement increases the PAV due to hyoid bone stretching. Hence, the resulting PAV enlargement effect is mainly produced at the level of the hypopharynx, so the procedure is not indicated to gain oropharyngeal volume [21]. On the other hand, the amount of chin advancement is limited to 10 mm due to two main aesthetic reasons: facial proportion harmony maintenance and the appearance of a visible step-off in the osteotomy line. Thus, the magnitude and direction of skeletal movements in OSA must be patient-tailored, depending on the underlying DFD, AHI, and PA morphology and the level of airway constriction/s. In other words, the surgical planning protocol must be adapted to the OSA requirements and PA enlargement without losing sight of occlusal and aesthetic parameters. In this context, adequate advancement and CCW rotation of the maxillomandibular complex (with chin advancement if required) is the gold standard protocol for OSA management and involves the same key points as in the UI-STP protocol [20].

15.6 Detrimental Skeletal Movements for the Airway

There is evidence to support significant narrowing of the PAV when the maxilla is moved downward or the facial skeletal framework is repositioned backward [22] (Fig. 15.4). In the first scenario, downward maxillary movement entails hyoid bone descent, which induces pull loss of the anterior pharyngeal wall. In the second scenario, backward movement of the maxillary and mandibular bones implies UA constriction due to backward positioning of the soft palate and base of the tongue, respectively.

Usually, maxillary downward movement is carried out in combination with other skeletal movements that counteract PAV narrowing through its enlargement. In the second case, some surgeons prescribe solely mandibular setback surgery for class III DFD. In such cases, potential postsurgical OSA must seriously be taken into consideration. From our point of view, in cases with severe skeletal class III DFD, CCW rotation combined with setback movement (if still required) should be considered instead of setback mandibular surgery alone, in order to avoid detrimental effects upon the airway. Moreover, double-jaw surgery with maxillary advancement should be considered to diminish the need for mandibular setback (Fig. 15.5). Thus, setback should be indicated only in specific cases, combined with CCW rotation and to a slight extent where PAV reduction might not induce OSA. According to our experience, mandibular setback only appears necessary in a minority of cases which are mostly coincident with cleft patients, hemimandibular elongation or hyperplasia, or underlying acromegaly. Similarly, among others, the management of Asian class III patients also may imply mandibular setback due to their characteristic inherent facial mid-third (and therefore nasal root and soft-tissue Nasion point) sagittal hypoplasia.

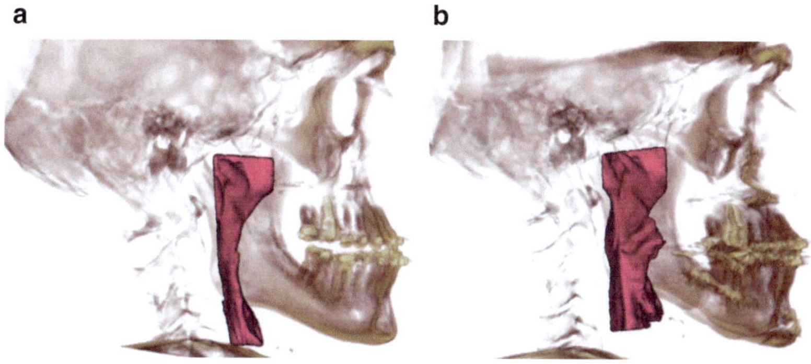

Fig. 15.5 (**a**) Initial airway evaluation of a class III case planned based on the Barcelona line reference (or UI-ST plane); and (**b**) postoperative airway evaluation where advancement of the maxillary bone and counterclockwise rotation of the maxillomandibular complex are carried out with proper aesthetic and occlusal results, and enlargement of the upper airway (instead of narrowing it when mandibular setback is performed)

15.7 Postoperative Follow-Up

Postoperative OSA clinical findings are monitored with PSG or home sleep apnea testing, the Epworth Sleepiness Scale, and CBCT. Monitoring is performed at two timepoints: at 1 month follow-up in order to quantify the impact of OS on the disease and at 1 year follow-up in order to rule out skeletal relapse as well as PAV relapse and, consequently, OSA recurrence. Overall, a mean skeletal relapse of 10% is to be expected, which is insufficient to offset the initial PAV gain [15].

15.8 Conclusions

To sum up, OS is the most effective and predictable surgical treatment option for patients diagnosed with moderate-to-severe OSA, although mild OSA cases also benefit from OS. Furthermore, when the UI-ST protocol as an absolute reference plane is used, mainly entailing advancement and CCW of the maxillomandibular framework, high success rates in terms of the occlusal, aesthetic, and enlargement of the pharyngeal airway/OSA cure endpoints are achieved.

However, further in-depth studies are required to obtain an algorithm of the amount and direction of skeletal movements required to enlarge specific levels of the UA. Moreover, further evidence is required to evaluate the impact of OS on young patients with mild OSA or without OSA but with a biretrusive facial profile in which ageing and soft-tissue loosening favor the development of OSA.

15.9 Key Points

- A multidisciplinary team is crucial to properly manage OSA patients.
- Orthognathic surgery is considered a curative treatment, since it increases the upper airway volume and reduces the apnea–hypopnea index.
- Current guidelines indicate orthognathic surgery for moderate and severe OSA patients, although those suffering from mild OSA also benefit from surgery.
- Patient-tailored orthognathic surgery should be carried out (instead of the classical standard 10 mm maxillomandibular advancement), keeping in mind both the facial and airway morphology of the patient.
- Maxillomandibular advancement with counterclockwise rotation provides more predictable airway expansive results.
- Mandibular advancement devices are reserved for non-obese patients with mild-to-moderate OSA refractory to or noncompliant with CPAP, and for patients who are not candidates for surgery due to health reasons, and also as a prognostic element in eventual orthognathic surgery.

References

1. Lloberes P, Durán-Cantolla J, Martínez-García MÁ, Marín JM, Ferrer A, Corral J, et al. Diagnosis and treatment of sleep apnea-hypopnea syndrome. Spanish Society of Pulmonology and Thoracic Surgery. Arch Bronconeumol. 2011;47(3):143–56.
2. Giralt-Hernando M, Valls-Ontañón A, Guijarro-Martínez R, Masià-Gridilla J, Hernández-Alfaro F. Impact of surgical maxillomandibular advancement upon pharyngeal airway volume and the apnoea-hypopnoea index in the treatment of obstructive sleep apnoea: systematic review and meta-analysis. BMJ Open Respir Res. 2019;6(1):1–13.
3. Durán J, Esnaola S, Rubio R, Iztueta A. Obstructive sleep apnoea-hypopnoea and related clinical features in a population-based sample of subjects aged 30 to 70 years. Am J Respir Crit Care Med [Internet]. 2001;163(3):685–9. Available from: http://www.ncbi.nlm.nih.gov/pubmed/11254524.
4. Kapur VK, Auckley DH, Chowdhuri S, Kuhlmann DC, Mehra R. Clinical practice guideline for diagnostic testing for adult obstructive sleep apnea: an American Academy of Sleep Medicine Clinical Practice Guideline. J Clin Sleep Med. 2017;13(3):479–504.
5. Posnick JC, Adachie A, Singh N, Choi E. "Silent" sleep apnea in dentofacial deformities and prevalence of daytime sleepiness after orthognathic and intranasal surgery. J Oral Maxillofac Surg [Internet]. 2018;76(4):833–43. https://doi.org/10.1016/j.joms.2017.09.003.
6. Schendel SA, Jacobson R, Khalessi S. Airway growth and development: a computerized 3-dimensional analysis. J Oral Maxillofac Surg [Internet]. 2012;70(9):2174–83. https://doi.org/10.1016/j.joms.2011.10.013.
7. Dicus Brookes CC, Boyd SB. Controversies in obstructive sleep apnea surgery. Oral Maxillofac Surg Clin North Am [Internet]. 2017;29(4):503–13. https://doi.org/10.1016/j.coms.2017.07.005.
8. Holty JEC, Guilleminault C. Maxillomandibular advancement for the treatment of obstructive sleep apnea: a systematic review and meta-analysis. Sleep Med Rev [Internet]. 2010;14(5):287–97. https://doi.org/10.1016/j.smrv.2009.11.003.
9. Jiang W, Bhattacharjee R, Nation J, Brigger MT. Completion of postoperative polysomnography for children with severe obstructive sleep apnea: a quality improvement project. Laryngoscope Investig Otolaryngol. 2022;7(July):1667–74.
10. Guilleminault C, Tilkian A, Dement WC. The sleep apnea syndromes. Annu Rev Med [Internet]. 1976;27(1):465–84. Available from: http://www.annualreviews.org/doi/10.1146/annurev.me.27.020176.002341.
11. Camacho M, Noller MW, Del Do M, Wei JM, Gouveia CJ, Zaghi S, et al. Long-term results for maxillomandibular advancement to treat obstructive sleep apnea: a meta-analysis. Otolaryngol Neck Surg [Internet]. 2019;142:019459981881515. https://doi.org/10.1177/0194599818815158.
12. Johns MW. A new method for measuring daytime sleepiness: the Epworth sleepiness scale. Sleep [Internet]. 1991;14(6):540–5. Available from: https://academic.oup.com/sleep/article-lookup/doi/10.1093/sleep/14.6.540.
13. Ramar K, Dort LC, Katz SG, Lettieri CJ, Harrod CG, Thomas SM, et al. Clinical practice guideline for the treatment of obstructive sleep apnea and snoring with oral appliance therapy: an update for 2015. J Clin sleep Med JCSM. 2015;11(7):773–827.
14. American Academy of Sleep Medicine. Evaluation, management and long-term care of OSA in adults clinical algorithm. Am Acad Sleep Med. 2015;August:1–6.
15. Giralt-Hernando M, Valls-Ontañón A, Haas Junior OL, Masià-Gridilla J, Hernández-Alfaro F. What are the surgical movements in orthognathic surgery that most affect the upper airways? A three-dimensional analysis. J Oral Maxillofac Surg. 2021;79(2):450–62.
16. Ayappa I, Rapoport DM. The upper airway in sleep: physiology of the pharynx. Sleep Med Rev. 2003;7(1):9–33.
17. Rubio-Bueno P, Landete P, Ardanza B, Vázquez L, Soriano JB, Wix R, et al. Maxillomandibular advancement as the initial treatment of obstructive sleep apnoea: is the mandibular occlusal plane the key? Int J Oral Maxillofac Surg. 2017;46(11):1363–71.
18. Hernández-Alfaro F, Vivas-Castillo J, de Oliveira RB, Haas Junior OL, Giralt-Hernando M, Valls-Ontañón A. Barcelona line. A multicenter validation study of a facial projection reference in orthognathic surgery. Br J Oral Maxillofac Surg [Internet]. 2022. Available from: https://www.sciencedirect.com/science/article/pii/S0266435622002819.;61:3.
19. Katz MI. Angle classification revisited 2: a modified Angle classification. Am J Orthod Dentofac Orthop. 1992;102(3):277–84.
20. Hernández-Alfaro F. Upper incisor to Soft Tissue Plane (UI-STP): a new reference for diagnosis and planning in dentofacial deformities. Med Oral Patol Oral Cir Bucal. 2010;15(5):8–10.
21. Chen K, Sun X, Wang L, Ni S, Wu Z, Gao Y, et al. A modified cosmetic genioplasty can affect airway space positively in skeletal class II patients: studying alterations of hyoid bone position and posterior airway space. Aesth Plast Surg. 2020;44(5):1639–55.
22. Gandedkar NH, Chng CK, Por YC, Yeow VKL, Ow ATC, Seah TE. Influence of bimaxillary surgery on pharyngeal airway in Class III deformities and effect on sleep apnea: a STOP-BANG questionnaire and cone-beam computed tomography study. J Oral Maxillofac Surg [Internet]. 2017;75(11):2411–21. https://doi.org/10.1016/j.joms.2017.05.028.

MIX
Papier aus verantwortungsvollen Quellen
Paper from responsible sources
FSC® C105338

If you have any concerns about our products,
you can contact us on
ProductSafety@springernature.com

In case Publisher is established outside the EU,
the EU authorized representative is:
Springer Nature Customer Service Center GmbH
Europaplatz 3, 69115 Heidelberg, Germany

Printed by Libri Plureos GmbH
in Hamburg, Germany